Essential
Sports Medicine

FIRST EDITION

Essential Sports Medicine

EDITED BY

Richard Higgins

Sports Physician
English Institute of Sport
Sheffield, UK
and Specialist in Sports and Musculoskeletal Medicine
and Sports Physician to Sheffield Wednesday Football Club

Bryan English

Sports Physician to Chelsea Football Club
Stamford Bridge
London, UK
and Specialist in Sports and Musculoskeletal Medicine

Peter Brukner

Associate Professor in Sports Medicine
Centre for Health, Exercise and Sports Medicine
Melbourne University
and Sports Physician
Olympic Park Sports Medicine Centre
Melbourne
Victoria, Australia

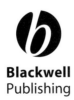

Blackwell
Publishing

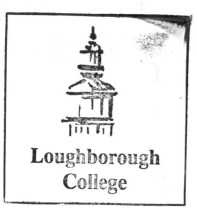

Loughborough College

© 2006 by Blackwell Publishing Ltd
Blackwell Publishing, Inc., 350 Main Street, Malden, Massachusetts 02148-5020, USA
Blackwell Publishing Ltd, 9600 Garsington Road, Oxford OX4 2DQ, UK
Blackwell Publishing Asia Pty Ltd, 550 Swanston Street, Carlton, Victoria 3053, Australia

The right of the Author to be identified as the Author of this Work has been asserted in accordance with the Copyright, Designs and Patents Act 1988.

First published 2006

Library of Congress Cataloging-in-Publication Data
Essential sports medicine / edited by Richard Higgins, Bryan English, Peter Brukner.
    p. ; cm.
   Includes index.
   ISBN-13: 978-1-4051-1438-7 (pbk.)
   ISBN-10: 1-4051-1438-X (pbk.)
   1. Sports medicine. 2. Sports injuries. I. Higgins, Richard, 1965-   . II. English, Bryan. III. Brukner, Peter, D.R.C.O.G.
   [DNLM: 1. Athletic Injuries -- rehabilitation. 2. Athletic Injuries --physiopathology. 3. Sports Medicine--methods. QT 261 E785 2005]
RC1210.E777 2005
617.1′027--dc22

20005016689

ISBN-13: 978-1-4051-1438-7
ISBN-10: 1-4051-1438-X

A catalogue record for this title is available from the British Library

Set in 9/12 Palatino by Sparks, Oxford – http://www.sparks.co.uk
Printed and bound in Harayana, India by Replika Press PVT Ltd

Commissioning Editor: Vicki Noyes
Editorial Assistant: Caroline Aders
Development Editor: Veronica Pock
Production Controller: Kate Charman

For further information on Blackwell Publishing, visit our website:
http://www.blackwellpublishing.com

Contents

Contributors

Editors

Richard Higgins
Sports Physician
English Institute of Sport
Coleridge Road
Sheffield, UK

Bryan English
Sports Physician to Chelsea
   Football Club
Stamford Bridge
London, UK

Peter Brukner
Associate Professor in Sports
   Medicine
Centre for Health, Exercise
   and Sports Medicine
University of Melbourne
Melbourne
Victoria, Australia

Contributors

Author of Chapter 16
Tom Adler
Evelyn Medical Centre
Derbyshire, UK

Author of Chapter 14
Mark E. Batt
Professor of Sports Medicine
Centre for Sports Medicine
Queens Medical Centre
Nottingham, UK

Author of Chapter 16
Phil Batty
Sports Physician to
   Blackburn Rovers Football
   Club
Blackburn
Lancashire, UK

Author of Chapter 5
Ian Beasley
Sports Physician to Arsenal
   Football Club
London, UK

Author of Chapter 10
Edwin van Beek
Professor in Radiology
Iowa University
Iowa, USA

Author of Chapter 16
Phillip Bell
Sports Physician and
   Medical Director of BUPA
   Wellness
London, UK

Author of Chapter 3
Pam Brown
The Grove Surgery
Uplands
Swansea, UK

Author of Chapter 13
Charlotte Cowey
Sports Physician to
   Tottenham Hotspur
   Football Club
London, UK

Author of Chapters 9 and 16
Bryan English
Sports Physician to Chelsea
   Football Club
London, UK

Author of Chapter 2
Mark Gillett
English Institute of Sport
   (EIS) Birmingham
Birmingham, UK

Author of Chapter 1

Bruce Hamilton
Cheif Medical Officer to UK
  Athletics
EIS Centre
Birmingham, UK

Author of Chapters 5, 6, 7, 8 and 17

Richard Higgins
Sports Physician
English Institute of Sport
Coleridge Road
Sheffield, UK

Author of Chapter 18

Dean Kenneally
Physiotherapist to Chelsea
  Football Club
Stamford Bridge
London, UK

Author of Chapter 16

Alistair Park
General Practitioner and
  Sports Physician
Oakhill Medical Centre
Oakhill Road
Dronfield
Derbyshire, UK

Author of Chapter 14

K. A. Strachan
GP and Sports Physician
Centre for Sports Medicine
Queens Medical Centre
Nottingham, UK

Author of Chapters 4 and 16

Simon Till
Consultant Rheumatologist
  and Sports Physician
Rheumatology Department
Royal Hallamshire Hospital
Sheffield, UK

Author of Chapter 11

John Walsh
Consultant Cardiologist
Division of Cardiovascular
  Medicine
Queen's Medical Centre,
  University Hospital
Nottingham, UK

Author of Chapters 12 and 15

Nick Webborn
Sports Physician
Sport's Life Ltd
Eastbourne
Sussex, UK

Author of Chapter 3

Jonathon Wheat
Sports Scientist
The Centre for Sports and
  Exercise Science
Sheffield Hallam University
Sheffield, UK

Author of Chapter 3

Edward M. Winter
Professor of Sports Science
The Centre for Sports and
  Exercise Science
Sheffield Hallam University
Sheffield, UK

Preface

Sports medicine has evolved beyond all recognition over the last decade. It has always provided an exciting, rewarding and challenging job, although some are discouraged due to a lack of career structure. Due to the tireless efforts of many, and most particularly Professor Mark Batt, sports and exercise medicine was granted speciality status earlier this year.

It is a fascinating area of medicine that will continue to grow and the aim of this book is to offer an initial insight into the subject for the medical student, GP or diploma student, or physiotherapist thinking of moving into this field.

The book has taken a number of years to compile due to its multi-author nature. Many sports medicine texts are written from a surgical viewpoint, but my intention was to produce a book written only by sports medicine practitioners, all at the forefront of their particular area of expertise.

I hope that this has been achieved, with almost every author in this book having had a significant influence on the specialism and many continuing to do so.

My two co-editors were also chosen as two of the figures that I feel have influenced not just my career but many others across the world. Professor Peter Brukner has headed the development of sports medicine both in Australia and around the world, and has become one of the most successful sports medicine authors with his text, *Clinical Sports Medicine*. Dr Bryan English has taken the role of the governing body medical officer to another level, working with UK athletics over three Olympic cycles before his recent move to Chelsea Football Club. His charisma and enthusiasm has helped bring together many sports physicians when he established the group UKADIS (United Kingdom Association of Doctors in Sport).

The passion for the subject demonstrated by those involved in this book has been a great motivating factor both for me and many others. I hope that this book will similarly stimulate such an interest in those who read it.

I'd finally like to thank Peter Davis who also helped steer me along this path at just the right time.

Richard Higgins, Sheffield, 2005

1 Medical issues and the role of the sports physician

Sports medicine is an increasingly popular field for medical practitioners, with specialized postgraduate courses (if not specialty recognition) now available in many countries. The practice of sports medicine requires skills in both general medical and musculoskeletal medicine in order to meet the needs of the modern athlete in the appropriate fashion.

The primary role of the sports physician is to maintain the athlete in a state of optimal health and well-being. This can only be achieved by ensuring that a close working relationship exists between members of the multidisciplinary team, for example, physiotherapy, orthopaedics, nutrition and massage (Fig. 1.1). The secondary role of the sports physician is to combine with the coaching and other support staff to assist in performance optimization. The conflict created between these two roles produces the difficult and unique environment in which the sports physician works.

The increased participation in exercise noted among the general public and the escalating professionalism/commercialization of elite sport, has highlighted the need for specialized medical practitioners, whilst also allowing those involved in sports medicine the opportunity of combining their passion for sport with their work.

Phillip Tissié may have been one of the first to practise 'sports medicine' when he described as 'toxic' the urine sample of an athlete who had just failed to break the world 24-hour cycling record in 1893; just 10 mL of the urine was required to kill a two-pound rabbit (24 hours later it took twice this

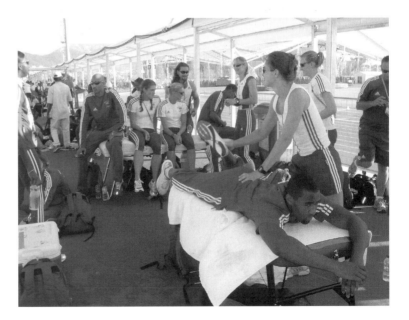

Fig. 1.1 The sports physician is required to work as part of a multidisciplinary team.

amount!). Perhaps ahead of his time, Tissié was opposed to elite competitive sport as it exists today, because of its potential dangers. Around the same time Charles-Edouard Brown-Séquard was undertaking experiments involving injections of testicular extracts, believing them to be the source of 'dynamogenic power', another issue that still haunts us in the 21st century. Sports physicians are now involved in all aspects of the care of both recreational and elite athletes, and are amongst the strongest advocates against the use of drugs in sport.

The aim of this chapter is to outline some of the roles and responsibilities of a sports physician, concentrating predominantly on the elite sports environment.

The team physician

An association with a successful, professional team is the goal of many sports physicians, and so it is important that they are able to work as part of a team, in which good communication between coaching staff and members of the multidisciplinary team is vital. Regular case conferences between clinical staff appear to be one of the most important processes to establish. Similarly, equally regular updates with coaching staff ensure that they are aware of ongoing concerns. Overriding this, however, are the concerns regarding confidentiality. While many teams will include a disclaimer, requiring athletes and doctors to disclose information, one must remember that first and foremost at all times is the welfare and consideration of the athlete (patient).

With this in mind it is imperative that the sports physician ensures that the correct environment is provided, with appropriately equipped private consulting rooms both protecting the athletes' confidentiality and maintaining their own professional standards and ethics.

Withdrawal of an athlete from competition is a key area, and it is important that the physician has previously clarified where the responsibility lies in this respect, so that he or she is comfortable making this decision, without being subject to external pressures.

Record-keeping is complicated by the fact that many consultations are undertaken not in the consulting room, but on the field or in the corridor. It goes without saying, however, that it is crucial that

clear and concise records are kept. The use of computerized records is growing and proving useful within this environment, with one of the major advantages being the ability to link to hand-held devices, allowing the physician to both access and record information 'in the field'.

Whereas general equipment requirements may vary, depending on squad size, the nature of the sport and the financial resources available, adequate access to emergency equipment is critical, with no compromise being acceptable (see Chapter 2).

It is not uncommon to find oneself entering a world that is filled with beliefs and treatment methods grounded in folklore. Difficulties may arise when these prove contrary to what is considered 'good medical practice', with tact and patience being required, while trying to establish one's position within a team.

Travelling with a team

International team travel can prove to be one of the most rewarding and challenging aspects to any sports physician's career. Demands may be high, with 24-hour cover often being required for several weeks at a time. It is helpful to divide the process into the following components: preparation, kit, travel and on-location care.

Preparation

A comprehensive history and examination should be undertaken prior to travelling, to ensure that the doctor is fully aware of any medical issues facing both athletes and staff. Accurate vaccination planning is facilitated by the production of both a detailed and timely travel itinerary. Vaccinations that should be considered as mandatory include:
- tetanus
- diphtheria
- measles
- mumps
- poliomyelitis
- rubella.

Those that should be considered on a more individualized basis (dependent on the nature of the sport, age of the individual, and location being visited) include:

- hepatitis A
- hepatitis B (important in contact sports)
- influenza
- malaria (oral prophylaxis)
- typhoid
- Japanese encephalitis
- cholera
- rabies
- meningococcus
- yellow fever.

Requirements are individually confirmed by consulting up-to-date guidelines.

Air travel

Circadian rhythms are the body's daily rhythms that are synchronized to the day/night cycle. Their control over the body's physiological and psychological systems affects many components of sports performance, producing daily variability in areas such as flexibility, power output and muscle strength.

The crossing of time zones can desynchronize these rhythms, leading to circadian dysrhythmia, or 'jet lag'. Jet-lag severity is directly proportional to the number of time zones crossed, and is heightened when flying eastwards. Symptoms include a disrupted sleep pattern, gastrointestinal disturbance, headaches and general malaise. It is estimated that it takes one day to readjust for each time zone crossed.

A number of simple strategies may help reduce symptoms:
- Adjusting one's sleeping pattern to that of the destination's time zone a few days before departure.
- Sleeping well on the night before departure.
- Minimizing time spent in transit with appropriate flight scheduling.
- Adjusting watches to the destination's local time on boarding.
- Use of relaxation techniques, ear plugs, and eye shields to assist in sleeping during and after the flight.

It has been suggested that following westward and eastward flights, competition should be arranged in the mornings and evenings, respectively, in order to optimize performance, by taking advantage of the circadian delay. Other means of minimizing jet lag include avoiding alcohol, regularly mobilizing in the aircraft cabin, and maintaining fluid and food intake. It is also proposed that eating a high-protein breakfast and a low-protein/high-carbohydrate dinner, following a time zone change, may assist in synchronization of rhythms.

The use of a short-acting hypnotic medication (e.g. temazepam) or melatonin may help in achieving sleep, therefore assisting in establishing a new circadian rhythm. Melatonin is a peptide secreted by the pineal gland that helps to induce sleep in conditions of low natural light. Although it has been shown to reduce the subjective symptoms of jet lag when taken before and after air travel, it must be used with care, so as not to upset further the body's circadian rhythm. As a result of the unpredictable individual effects, and the potential for prolonged drowsiness, the British Olympic Association Medical Committee advises against the use of hypnotics or melatonin in international travel. Under no circumstances should hypnotic medication or melatonin be used for the first time before a major competition.

On arrival one should evaluate the infection risk in relation to sanitation levels and insect vectors. Any doubts regarding the water supply are an immediate indicator for the use of sealed, bottled water for drinking and oral hygiene. Similarly, ice cubes, salads or other foods washed in tap water, should be avoided. In these circumstances the general rule of 'cook it, peel it or leave it alone', should be applied. Drink bottles should be regularly cleaned, with bottled water, especially if sports drinks are being used. A brush should be taken for this purpose.

Mosquitoes are responsible not only for the transmission of the parasites that cause malaria, but also for arboviruses causing dengue fever, yellow fever and Japanese encephalitis. The use of light-coloured long-sleeved clothing, insect repellents and sleeping nets is recommended in high-risk areas. Antimalarial prophylaxis varies depending on location, duration of stay and an individual's medical history.

Heat acclimatization can take up to two weeks, and until this is achieved, performance may be impaired. The volume and intensity of training should be reduced on arrival, with a gradual increase over the next two weeks, whilst also progressing from the cooler to the warmer times of the day. Fluid intake should increase, with body weight and urine volume being used to monitor adequate replacement.

Light-coloured loose-fitting clothing and sun block should be worn to minimize the risk of heat-related illness.

Travelling from sea level to compete at altitude requires a similar period of acclimatization, the alternative being to compete within 24 hours of arrival.

On returning from international team travel, it is important that a clear and concise report is produced for the team management, including an assessment of all aspects of the tour, being careful, however, not to breach confidentiality. Medical reports of all athletes seen should be forwarded to the appropriate physician or general practitioner.

The medical bag

The contents of a medical bag will depend on the nature of the sport, the availability of auxiliary medical services, and the number of athletes involved. As a general rule no prohibited medications should be included, to prevent the possibility of accidental and inappropriate use. When covering events it is useful to carry a small kit containing essential contents at all times, whilst keeping a more significant kit handy on the sideline.

The following aims to provide a system for considering the contents of any medical bag, but is not intended to be exhaustive.

1 Emergency equipment
  • Multi-size hard collar
  • Airway devices (oropharyngeal, nasopharyngeal)
  • Intravenous access, giving sets and fluids
  • Resuscitation equipment (bag/mask, automated external defibrillator (AED))
  • Spinal board
  • Emergency medications
2 Medications
  • Upper respiratory tract (URT):
    – decongestants;
    – asthma medication;
    – ear drops;
    – nasal drops;
    – throat sprays/lozenges.
  • Eye drops:
    – antibiotic, anaesthetic, antihistamine, natural tears;
  • Antibiotics (various broad spectrum)
  • Gastrointestinal:
    – antidiarrhoeals;
    – laxatives;
    – antispasmodics;
    – antacids;
    – antiemetics.
  • Cardiovascular:
    – emergency medication;
    – glyceryl trinitrate spray.
  • Analgesics and anti-inflammatories:
    – paracetamol;
    – codeine;
    – NSAIDs.
  • Cortisone (injectable)
  • Long- and short-acting local anaesthetic (injectable)
  • Skin creams (cortisone, antihistamine, antibiotic, sunscreens)
3 Suture equipment
  • Including local anaesthetic (with and without adrenaline)
  • Steristrips
4 Sharps bin
5 Variable needles, syringes
6 Dressings (dry, moist, nonstick)
7 Alcohol, Betadine swabs
8 Medical equipment
  • Otoscope/ophthalmoscope
  • Sphygmomanometer
  • Stethoscope
  • Mirror
  • Thermometer
  • Glucometer
  • Nebulizer
  • Peak flow monitor
9 Dental kit
10 Ice bags
11 Sterile/nonsterile gloves
12 Multiple tapes
13 Prescription pad, headed notepaper.

Common medical conditions

Asthma and the athlete

Presentation

Asthma is a common condition affecting up to 10% of the population. Presenting symptoms are of intermittent wheeze, shortness of breath, chest tightness, and a persistent cough. Asthmatics can be categorized as atopic, classical, or exercise induced. Exercise-induced asthma (EIA) is characterized by symptoms during or after exercise, and while up to 80% of true asthmatics will suffer symptoms of EIA, it may also occur in otherwise healthy individuals.

EIA refers to the transient narrowing of the airways that occurs following approximately 6–8 minutes of moderately intense activity. Its occurrence can compromise performance and prolong recovery from exercise. This condition is increasingly recognized by the medical fraternity but often not by the athlete; some figures would suggest that as many as 23% of Olympic athletes may suffer from EIA.

With continuous exercise in cold, dry air being the most common trigger, sports such as running, cross-country skiing and ice skating are frequently associated with the condition. High levels of atmospheric pollution or allergens are also common aggravants.

Two hypotheses have been used to attempt to explain this response of transient bronchospasm following exercise. The thermal hypothesis suggests 'airway cooling' followed by rapid rewarming as causation. This theory, however, has largely been discredited. By contrast, there is mounting evidence supporting the osmotic hypothesis, which proposes that initial dehydration, followed by increases in osmolarity, leading to mast cell degranulation and release of mediators, may precipitate EIA.

Diagnosis
The diagnosis may be made in several ways, the simplest being a clinical trial with an inhaled bronchodilator. With a history suggestive of asthma, an improvement in both symptoms and peak expiratory flow rate (PEFR) of approximately 15% following the treatment provides a presumptive diagnosis. The use of an exercise challenge is similarly practical, involving exercising at an intensity just below anaerobic threshold for 10–12 minutes, with PEFR measurements being taken pre-exercise, then 1, 3, 6, 10 and 15 minutes following exercise. The various testing methods used to achieve a diagnosis of EIA are described in Chapter 17.

Management
Education of the athlete is important, and an 'asthma action plan' should be designed for each individual to give them the confidence and ability to manage exacerbations. Regular testing of pulmonary function will allow an athlete and coach objectively to assess the relationship of lung function to performance. Environmental manipulation, for instance running with a mask in cool air, using a humidifier when training indoors, nose breathing, and avoiding exercising in polluted air, can assist in minimizing the severity of EIA; however, in reality these suggestions are often impractical. One method of reducing symptoms is by the induction of a 'refractory period', by using a steady, prolonged warm-up, to avoid inducing bronchospasm during this exercise phase, thus allowing vigorous exercise to follow without the production of symptoms. This period will often allow further symptom-free exercise sessions to be undertaken over the next 2–4 hours. It appears, however, that only 50% of athletes become refractory, so this will not work for all.

Pharmacological management comprises the use of β_2-agonists (salbutamol), taken either once or twice, 15–30 minutes before exercise. Long-acting β_2-agonists (salmeterol) have also proved beneficial if a prolonged duration of coverage is required. It is important to note that both the World Anti-Doping Agency (WADA) and the International Olympic Committee (IOC) restricts the use of β_2-agonists, requiring formal documentary evidence of their requirement.

Mast cell stabilizers (sodium cromoglycate) and leukotriene receptor antagonists may also be useful. The use of inhaled corticosteroids should be continued, in order to minimize airway inflammation in the management of classical asthma and refractory EIA.

Treatment failure may be the result of a number of factors such as drug dosage, empty canisters, and drug inhalation technique. A continued lack of response to treatment may suggest misdiagnosis or possible secondary gain.

Treatment of the acute, severe asthma attack 'on the field' involves the administration of bronchodilator therapy (e.g. salbutamol) followed by immediate transportation to a medical facility. If a nebulizer or oxygen is available then they should be utilized, otherwise spacer devices may assist in the more effective delivery of inhaled medications.

Epilepsy

Presentation

Epilepsy is characterized by recurrent seizure activity, the result of abnormal electrical discharge within the cortical and subcortical neurones of the brain. True epilepsy may affect up to 3% of the population, with most presentations occurring before the age of 30. The majority of epileptic seizures are idiopathic in nature; however, pathological events may be responsible: for instance, stroke, infection or neoplasm of the central nervous system, metabolic derangement, birth trauma, or rarely anatomical abnormalities associated with conditions such as Sturge–Weber syndrome.

Seizures may be preceded by an aura, for instance a peculiar taste or smell, which is usually of a similar nature on each occasion. Drowsiness, headache and fatigue are common following an epileptic seizure, but except in this immediate post-ictal phase, examination of a patient with epilepsy is usually normal.

Management

Up to 80% of individuals with epilepsy can be controlled on a single drug. Many of these medications, however, can produce drowsiness and visual disturbance and so their side-effect profile must be carefully considered before making exercise recommendations. Although drug efficacy has not been found to be affected by activity, sudden changes in weight or body composition as a result of training may affect serum levels, which should therefore be monitored closely.

Although seizure frequency is reduced during exercise, it increases in the immediate postexercise phase. It has been postulated that this is a direct result of the increase in concentration of gamma-aminobutyric acid (GABA) during exercise, suppressing electrical activity within the brain.

Well-controlled epilepsy should have no effect on an athlete's performance; however, during the post-ictal phase (which may last up to a few days) performance may be affected by fatigue and impaired alertness, balance and coordination. Similarly, as previously mentioned, anticonvulsant medication may impair cognitive function, vision, concentration and coordination, all of which are important in exercise and sport performance.

Athletes who are seizure free and are well controlled on medication, have few contraindications to sport. However, some activities are associated with unacceptable risk, should a seizure occur, and consequently are contraindicated for people with epilepsy. Absolute contraindications include sports such as rock climbing, scuba diving, flying, hang gliding, parachuting, shooting, archery and boxing. Relative contraindications include swimming and water sports, cross-country skiing, back packing, cycling, skating, horse riding, gymnastics, motor sports and many contact sports.

Additionally there are a number of physiological extremes, commonly encountered in competitive sport, that may precipitate seizure activity (e.g. fatigue, sleep deprivation, hypoxia, hyponatraemia, hyperthermia, hypoglycaemia) and these situations should be avoided where possible.

Concussion

Concussion is defined as 'a clinical syndrome characterized by immediate and transient post-traumatic impairment of neural function, such as alteration of consciousness, disturbance of vision and/or equilibrium'. The important words in this description are 'immediate and 'transient', that is, the symptoms and signs of concussion are neither delayed nor persistent.

In recent years there has been an increase in the use of headgear and mouth guards with a view to preventing concussive head injuries, which are a significant problem in contact sports. It has been shown, however, that the risk of concussion is unlikely to be reduced by the use of this commercially available headgear. Interestingly, it has also been shown that players wearing headgear perceived increased levels of safety and hence an ability to tackle more forcefully. Although mouth guards do offer protection against dental injury, there is little evidence that they offer any protection against concussion. In short, the prevention of concussion and other head injury, is best achieved by education and the enforcement of appropriate rules preventing dangerous play.

Diagnosis

A variety of symptoms may present following injury, such as loss of consciousness (LOC), memory disturbance, headache, nausea, poor coordination, dizziness, double/blurred vision, and confusion. Additionally, the athlete may present with a vacant stare and delayed verbal responses and actions. Importantly, loss of consciousness is not a prerequisite, and memory disturbance is the only pathognomonic symptom.

It has been found that a series of questions aimed at evaluating recent memory were more sensitive than using long-term recall in achieving a diagnosis. Examples of these questions are:

- Which ground are we at?
- Which quarter/half is it?
- How far into the quarter is it? The first, middle, or last 10 minutes?
- Which side scored last?
- Which team did we play last week?
- Did we win last week.
- 'Serial sevens'.

The assessment of concussion severity has traditionally involved measurement of the duration of post-traumatic amnesia and loss of consciousness (e.g. Cantu and Colorado Grading Systems). However, the validity of this approach is unknown, as these systems are based on little scientific evidence.

On-field assessment of concussion involves first aid, with a careful primary review for associated injuries, such as to the cervical spine (see Chapter 2).

Management

Once a patient has been stabilized and removed from the field of play, assessment should continue in the quiet of the dressing room. A detailed history and neurological examination, including serial assessment of recent memory function, should be performed. If a player has any symptoms or signs of concussion, then that player should not be allowed to return to play, should not be left alone, and should be reviewed at regular intervals by medical personnel.

Certain situations require additional caution, for instance, a concussional injury in children and adolescents, which may also be associated with an increased risk of diffuse brain swelling, known as second impact syndrome (note: there continues to be some debate about the existence and prevalence of this diagnosis). Urgent referral should also be sought following concussive incidents where there is any suspicion of a cervical spine fracture, focal neurology, prolonged LOC or confusion, or a significant medical history. Discharge home should only be allowed under the supervision of a mature adult, with instructions on how to manage any deterioration in symptoms.

Most recognized 'return-to-play' guidelines are based on injury severity grading systems; however, many of these systems are not based on sound scientific research. Mandatory exclusion criteria, based on a particular grade of injury, are inherently dangerous in that they may lead to under-reporting of concussive events or allow a premature return to play. In the days following a concussive incident, regular symptom assessment and examination should be performed. Examination should include neuropsychological testing. More recently, computerized assessment packages have become popular and are increasingly utilized in professional sport. On return of the neuropsychological testing to baseline levels and with no symptoms at rest, the athlete is allowed to perform light aerobic exercise. When managed without any return of symptoms, the athlete can progress to noncontact drills, finally returning to contact training, before being allowed to return to play. Persistence of, or deterioration in symptomatology warrants further investigation by a neurologist or sports physician.

Further reading

Maddocks DL, Dicker GD, Saling MM *et al.* The assessment of orientation following concussion in athletes. *Clin J Sport Med* 1995, **5**(1), 32–5.

2 Acute care

This chapter will focus on the emergency aspects of acute assessment and treatment required to work safely as a pitch-side healthcare professional. The acute management of soft tissue injuries is covered elsewhere in this book.

Equipment

The level of training and experience of the sports physician becomes irrelevant if the essential equipment required for immediate care is not available. The following items should be readily to hand (Fig. 2.1):
• Oropharyngeal airways (OPAs)
• Nasopharyngeal airways (NPAs)
• A pocket mask
• Semi-rigid cervical spine collars
• A spinal board complete with suitable immobilization strapping
• A portable oxygen cylinder complete with both a non-rebreathing (trauma) mask and a bag-valve mask attachment
• An automated external defibrillator.
Other items such as a handheld suction device and a scoop stretcher are highly desirable.

Some may view this list as ambitious, but it encompasses only the minimum equipment necessary to safely treat an unconscious athlete on the field of play. Furthermore, in sports such as the equestrian events and cycling where higher velocity trauma may be anticipated, a more extensive array of equipment will be required.

Approaching the injured athlete

Scene safety must be assured before attending the casualty. This usually entails either stopping play or having marshalls divert oncoming runners or riders away from the treatment area. In the heat of the moment this necessity can easily be forgotten, putting the safety of the attending medic at risk.

The primary survey

This technique is now universally taught on resuscitation courses and is based on the ABCDE principle (Box 2.1). It provides a structured approach to acute assessment and ensures that those problems that

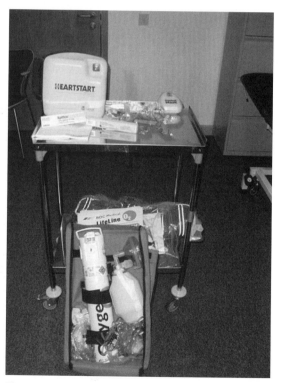

Fig. 2.1 Emergency equipment requirements.

Box 2.1 The primary survey

Airway with C spine protection
Breathing
Circulation
Disability
Exposure/Environment

Box 2.2 Airway assessment and indicators of airway patency

Airway assessment

- LOOK: at the mouth and face for deformity and for the chest to rise and fall with breathing.
- FEEL: for breath on the side of your face.
- LISTEN: for breath sounds at the casualty's mouth.

Clinical indicators of airway patency

- Talking normally → airway clear.
- Gurgling → fluid partially obstructing airway.
- Snoring → soft tissue partially obstructing airway.
- Stridor → upper airway partial obstruction, e.g. teeth or gumshield.
- No breath sounds felt or heard → complete airway obstruction.

---

may be life threatening are treated in an appropriate time order.

Airway assessment with cervical spine control

Assessment of airway patency should be performed simultaneously with manual in-line stabilization (MILS) of the neck, until a cervical spine injury can be reliably excluded. Ideally an assistant should maintain the neck in a neutral position while the medic evaluates the airway. If an assistant is not available then the medic can perform MILS and perform a jaw thrust manoeuvre from the head end if it is required. Box 2.2 summarizes the stages of airway assessment and the implications of clinical findings.

Methods of opening the airway

The standard techniques used to open a partially obstructed airway are:
- Head tilt-chin lift (Fig. 2.2)
- Jaw thrust (Fig. 2.3).

In situations where a cervical spine injury cannot be excluded, jaw thrust is the manoeuvre of choice because it requires less movement of the cervical vertebrae.

If these techniques fail to open the airway, consideration can then be given to using an OPA if the

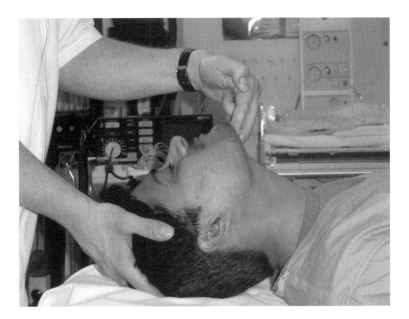

Fig. 2.2 Head tilt-chin lift.

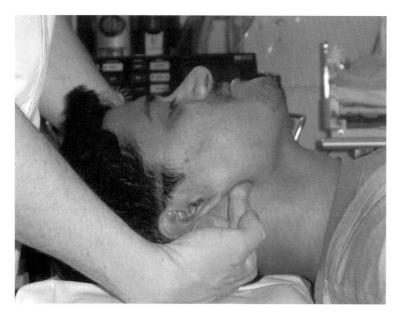

Fig. 2.3 Jaw thrust.

casualty is unconscious, or an NPA if the patient is semiconscious.

Breathing assessment

In practice, breathing and airway are assessed simultaneously. Box 2.3 outlines the key points essential for the clinical evaluation of breathing.

Circulatory assessment

The two major clinical tools used are:
• A capillary refill time of less than 2 seconds
• Pulse rate and volume.
It must be remembered that in a young person at least 1500 mL of blood, or 30% of the circulatory vol-

ume, will have to be lost in order to produce a fall in systolic blood pressure. Hence in the majority of cases of trauma in sport, blood pressure assessment is not an immediate priority. Box 2.4 gives a guide to the minimum likely systolic blood pressure associated with the three major palpable pulses.

Disability assessment

Disability in reality refers to a gross neurological assessment, which has two components:
• Pupillary size and response to light
• AVPU score (outlined in Box 2.5).

Exposure and environment

The injured athlete should be exposed to reveal the extent of the injury, mindful that overexposure to the spectators and media should be prevented by appropriate means. The ambient environment should also

---

Box 2.3 Clinical evaluation of breathing

• LOOK: for equal chest movement on both sides and any wounds over the chest wall. Unequal movement may indicate a pneumothorax, haemothorax, rib fractures or a flail chest.
• FEEL: for a central trachea, neck swelling, surgical emphysema of the neck or chest and palpable rib or laryngeal fractures.
• LISTEN: for bilaterally equal breath sounds and chest wall percussion note on both sides.

Box 2.4 Minimum likely systolic blood pressures for major pulses

Carotid pulse: systolic BP > 60 mmHg
Femoral pulse: systolic BP > 70 mmHg
Radial pulse: systolic BP > 80 mmHg

> **Box 2.5** The 'AVPU' disability assessment
>
> Alert: able to obey commands.
> Verbalizing: talking but incoherent or irrational.
> Pain: responding to painful stimuli.
> Unresponsive: no response to any stimulus.

be considered, as a severely injured player will have impaired adaptations to climatic variation.

The principles of the primary survey

The rescuer should not progress through the algorithm unless the preceding element has been secured. For example, if the rescuer identifies a complete airway obstruction but moves on to assess the pulse rate before clearing the airway, the patient will probably die from hypoxia regardless of his or her circulatory status.

Continual reassessment of the ABC is vital to identify deterioration of cardio-respiratory status at the earliest opportunity.

The secondary survey

This refers to the detailed assessment of the casualty undertaken after the 'time-critical functions' of the primary survey have been assessed and stabilized. In most cases of onfield injury, the secondary survey will be performed either after the player has been moved to a designated area or after transfer to hospital.

Advanced life support

The three major rhythms encountered in cardiac arrest are asystole, pulseless electrical activity and ventricular fibrillation (VF). Of these VF carries by far the best prognosis, provided that defibrillation takes place at the earliest opportunity. Statistically the chances of successful defibrillation decrease by about 10% for every minute that passes after the VF arrest. For this reason it is imperative that a defibrillator is readily available at sports events. At major events, the paramedic crew in attendance will carry a defibrillator; however, at smaller events a paramedic crew will not legally be required, providing the medic and the sporting organization with a predicament. In the past, automated external defibrillators (AEDs) were considered too expensive for many smaller organizations to buy, but over the last few years the purchase price has decreased dramatically, making AEDs increasingly accessible. The medic and the sports organization employing his or her services must reach an agreement as to whether the clinical risk justifies the financial outlay. The risk involved will obviously vary according to the age of the sporting population in question. It is important to dismiss the misapprehension that effective basic life support (BLS) will suffice until a defibrillator becomes available. Although training in BLS techniques is vital for medics covering sports events, effective BLS will not produce a change in cardiac rhythm for a patient in VF.

Further training

A variety of courses exist that cater for both the healthcare professional and members of the public who wish to learn BLS skills. Courses are only of use if the individuals concerned continually practise and update the skills pertinent to their occupation and specific sporting environment.

CHAPTER 3

3 Sport and exercise science

Introduction

Interest in mechanisms that explain rather than simply describe performance has a long history and can be traced to at least the time of Hippocrates and the ancient Olympic Games. The emperor Marcus Aurelius (121–180 AD), for instance, had schools in Rome that were designed to improve the training and hence performance of gladiators. However, the concerted appliance of scientific principles to sport and exercise, characterized by the randomized controlled trial, accelerated at the beginning of the last century when A.V. Hill began his extraordinary career in the physiology of exercise.

In the 1930s the coach Gerschler and the cardiologist Reindel combined to develop interval training, which they used to good effect with German middle-distance runners, notably Rudolf Harbig. Pugh's work in connection with the ascent of Everest in 1953 contributed much to our knowledge and understanding of how the body uses oxygen, and Franz Stampfl working with (Sir) Roger Bannister cemented the need for a scientific approach to training.

This science is formalized academically in the UK through undergraduate and postgraduate training in institutes of higher education. Academic programmes in universities were introduced in 1976 and now some 10 000 students graduate each year with sport and exercise-related degrees. The application of academic skills is recognized as an essential part of sport by bodies such as UK Sport and the British Olympic Association. The British Association of Sport and Exercise Sciences, formed in 1984, is the lead body for sport and exercise science in the UK and is both a learned society and a professional body for sport and exercise scientists.

It is now recognized that distinction can be made between two broad groupings, although there are elements common to both: first, those whose aspirations are competitive and for whom improvements in performance have the primary aim of success in competition; and second, those whose interests are health oriented and for whom exercise is recreational. Sport and exercise science applies to both.

The three major contributing disciplines in this science are biomechanics, physiology and psychology. This chapter will focus on the contributions of the first two. In biomechanics the emphasis will be on technique and injury prevention, while in physiology the emphasis will be on mechanisms that underpin performance.

The physiology of exercise

The physiology of exercise is the study of how the body responds and adapts to exercise. Exercise does not necessarily involve movement, as instanced by the Maltese Cross in gymnastics, the scrum in both codes of rugby, and fine skills required in activities like archery and shooting. However, the ability to perform exercise depends on effective force production by muscle that has to be coordinated. This coordination could be for exercise that is short duration and high intensity, such as sprinting, or for exercise that is long duration and low intensity, characterized by endurance events. In between these two are what have been termed the multiple-sprint activities in which high-intensity or even all-out exercise is interspersed with periods of relative recovery. Many sports are of this type, including such field games as association football, rugby and hockey; racket sports such as squash, tennis and badminton; and court games such as netball, basketball and volleyball.

Muscle and exercise

The three types of muscle involved are skeletal (also known as striated or voluntary), smooth (also known as involuntary) and cardiac, which has inbuilt rhythmicity. Irrespective of the type, the function of muscle is to exert force but the precise outcome of stimulation is still the subject of debate. For simplicity, three types of activity can be considered: concentric, in which a muscle shortens during its force development; eccentric, when it lengthens during such development; and isometric, in which muscle length remains the same. This gives rise to a useful definition of exercise that applies both in sport and exercise: exercise is a potential disruption to homeostasis by muscle activity that is either exclusively or in combination, concentric, eccentric or isometric.

Fitness

The capability to perform exercise depends on a variety of factors other than those that are purely physiological or mechanical. Mental skills, the size, shape and composition of the body, and even aspects such as opportunity to take part in activities all contribute. A key challenge is to provide children especially with these opportunities, so that talent can be identified and appropriately nurtured. Moreover, there are health benefits to be gained from an active lifestyle, as evidenced by worrying trends that diseases related to a sedentary lifestyle are increasing as children become less active, with these effects becoming more evident in later life.

Energetics: adenosine triphosphate (ATP)

The ability to perform exercise is determined fundamentally by the availability of the body's energy currency, adenosine triphosphate (ATP). It is imperative that an energy crisis is avoided, and that the body's demands for energy can be matched by provision. Clearly there comes a point when the crisis occurs; the ability to delay its onset is a defining feature of the champion athlete. Table 3.1 illustrates the endogenous stores of the high-energy phosphagens, and it is striking just how modest these endogenous stores are. What is crucial is the body's ability to resynthesize ATP, and it is these resynthesis mechanisms that have a major influence on the ability to perform exercise.

It was thought that the resynthesis mechanisms ran in a progressive order. For instance, that anaerobic provision by way of lactic acid only occurred when phosphocreatine was depleted. We now know that each of the mechanisms probably runs in parallel along a continuum in which it is simply the emphasis that changes.

Aerobic energy provision and the Fick equation

In 1890, Adolf Fick presented an equation that recognized the interrelationships between cardiovascular, cardiopulmonary and peripheral function:

Table 3.1 Endogenous energy stores in humans

Store	Muscular concentration (mmol/kg)		Energy·M^{-1} (kJ)	Total energy (kJ) in humans (assuming a body mass of 75 kg and a muscle mass of 20 kg)
	Wet	Dry		
ATP	5	25	42	4
CP	17	70	44	15
Glycogen	80	–	2900	4600
Fat	–	–	10 000	30 000

ATP, adenosine triphosphate; CP, creatine phosphate.

$$Vo_2 = Q \times a - VO_2$$

where Vo_2 = oxygen uptake (L/min), Q = cardiac output (L/min), $a - VO_2$ = arterio-venous oxygen difference (mL/100 mL blood). This equation encapsulates the tripartite nature of oxygen uptake, namely extraction of oxygen from the atmosphere by the lung, transport by the cardiovascular system and utilization by muscle. The maximum rate at which an athlete can extract, transport and utilize oxygen, that is their Vo_2max, strongly influences their ability to perform endurance-type exercise and reduces their dependence on anaerobic metabolism. The precise point where this dependence becomes marked, the anaerobic threshold, has been the topic of enthusiastic debate for nearly 30 years but it can safely be said that if an athlete has a high Vo_2max and can operate at a high proportion of this maximum without resorting to anaerobic metabolism, they are probably exceedingly capable endurance performers.

The Vo_2max is probably limited by cardiac output because it has been demonstrated that muscle can use more oxygen than it receives. The experiments that were undertaken to demonstrate this have allegedly given rise to the use of blood reinfusions to increase oxygen handling capabilities and latterly, the use of erythropoietin (see Chapter 17).

Physiological basis of training

The aim of training is to bring about an adaptation, and the basic model is illustrated in Fig. 3.1. This model applies at all levels of biological organization: to the whole body; the body's systems; organs; tissues; cells; and, fundamentally, subcellular proc-

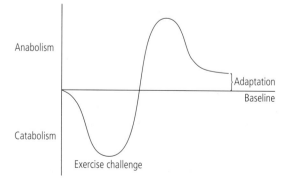

Fig. 3.1 Yakovlev's model of adaptation.

esses. Moreover, it also applies to phases of training, also known as cycles. These cycles could be short term, for example over 3 days, say, or mescycles, which could last for weeks or even months.

There are three main parts to this model: first, the exercise challenge, which has a catabolic effect; second, recovery during which anabolism takes place; and third, adaptation, which is represented as a rise in baseline function. Each of these has to be balanced carefully to ensure a progression that fully capitalizes on the athlete's potential, whilst not resulting in an incomplete or even maladaptive response, characterized by unexplained underperformance syndromes. The exercise challenge has to provide an overload that presents a stimulus greater than that usually experienced. This has to be followed by recovery to allow adaptive mechanisms to occur and, in the case, say, of nutrition, allow adequate time for replacement. If the challenge and recovery are mismatched, instead of there being a gradual increase in performance, the outcome can be a gradual decline.

A key development of the last decade has been the Human Genome Project, in which the detailed makeup of human chromosomes and their inherent genes has been unravelled. This has exciting implications for our understanding both of protein synthesis and the control of tissue. It has also raised the spectre of genetic engineering of athletes to accompany the blight that is drug abuse in sport. Time will tell whether developments are beneficial or otherwise.

Overtraining (unexplained underperformance syndromes, UUPS)

A distressing feature that can accompany demanding training programmes is, over a period of weeks, a gradual deterioration of performance, which can be made worse by harder training. This downward trend, explained in outline by the supercompensation model that was considered earlier, is not easy to detail because there are several possible mechanisms. Evidence suggests that the deterioration is related to volume rather than intensity.

One mechanism could be simply inadequate diet; the athlete does not consume enough carbohydrate so intramuscular concentrations of glycogen fall. A brief reduction in intensity and volume of training accompanied by high-carbohydrate meals can quickly reverse the condition. More troublesome are instances in which autoimmune function is compromised. These can be characterized by increased incidences of upper respiratory tract infections, or post-viral syndromes, the later being much more difficult to prove or quantify scientifically. Other metabolic conditions can of course be responsible. Whatever the cause, diagnosis and management require close working relationships between the clinician and the sport and exercise scientist, in close conjunction with the athlete and coach.

Sport and exercise biomechanics

Biomechanics is generally considered to be the application of mechanical principles to living organisms. More specifically, it was defined as the science that examines forces acting on and within a biological structure and their effects. Sport and exercise biomechanics is, therefore, the application of biomechanical principles to sport and exercise. Generally, sport and exercise biomechanics has two main aims: to improve performance and reduce the risk of injury. There is much research in each area but this section will focus specifically on injury. Approaches in sport and exercise biomechanics comprise kinematic and kinetic analyses. Kinematic approaches measure variables that describe movement without reference to the forces responsible, whereas kinetic analyses do examine the forces that in the human body, for example, cause or restrict motion. Here, the focus will be on kinematic analysis. Moreover, only overuse injuries will be considered.

Sport- and exercise-related injuries

It has been estimated that of all cases attending an accident and emergency department in the UK, 10% are due to sports injury. In addition, it is forecast that 10% of all sports injuries will result in absence from work, highlighting the deleterious effect on the nation's economy. These facts support the need for sports injuries to be taken seriously by practitioners and athletes alike. Overuse injuries result from repetitive traumas that are below the single event injury threshold, preventing tissue from self-repair and so producing a combined fatigue effect over time.

Approximately half of all sports injuries are overuse rather than traumatic in nature, and these injuries such as Achilles tendinosis, are dealt with in detail in the relevant sports injury sections of this book.

Specific examples

Perhaps surprisingly, few strong links have been established between movements or techniques in sport or exercise and specific injuries. However, two such links that are often cited are the association between lower back injury in cricket fast bowlers and the 'mixed' bowling technique, and the effects of rugby scrummaging on neck and spinal injuries. As regards the association between lower back injury and the 'mixed' bowling technique, several injury risk factors are present. The mixed technique involves a combination of the front-on and side-on actions. At rear-foot impact the shoulders face obliquely across the pitch but during the delivery stride, the shoulders counter-rotate to produce a shoulder alignment typical of a side-on action. It is this shoulder counter-rotation that is one of the kinematic factors linked to lower back injury; six of 17 mixed bowlers were reported as having stress fractures of the lumbar spine, and seven demonstrated soft tissue injury.

Running injuries

Such strong links have not been found in other sport and exercise movements such as running. Approximately 32 million North Americans include running as part of their exercise regime. As many as 65% of all runners will sustain an overuse injury during the first year of running that will cause them either to seek medical attention or to stop running either temporarily or even permanently. These worrying figures alone highlight the need to study the factors related to the high injury rate in runners.

Injuries to the lower extremity predominate in running. Of these injuries, most are overuse, and several aetiological factors, such as excessive pronation, have been implicated. During the normal gait cycle the foot strikes the ground in a supinated position, then pronates until approximately 50% of the stance phase, before supinating once more until take-off. Pronation allows the impact forces to be absorbed over a longer period by the supporting structures of the leg and thereby reduces the effective magnitude of these forces. Lack of pronation is problematic because the supporting structures have to absorb the shock loads abruptly. Despite the benefits of normal pronation, excessive subtalar pronation has been linked with several running-related injuries, particularly those of the knee, though with little experimental evidence. Reasons for this uncertainty include the probable multifactorial nature of these injuries and ethical constraints, which prevent prospective trials in which injury is an intended outcome. Figure 3.2 represents the interaction between intrinsic and extrinsic factors associated with injury, proposing that provided the cumulative effects both of the intrinsic and extrinsic factors remain below hypothetical threshold values, the runner will remain injury free.

Recent developments in running injury research

The focus of many running injury studies to date has been the action of lower extremity joints individually rather than the interaction or coupling between the joints. It is clear that the actions of these joints are linked and consideration of the interactions and coupling is warranted. Indeed, a proposed mechanism for injuries in running is an asynchrony, or timing discrepancy, between subtalar and knee joint actions throughout the running stride. Both subtalar pronation and knee flexion promote internal rotation of the tibia. Conversely, subtalar supination and knee extension promote external rotation of the tibia. The transitions of knee joint flexion to extension and subtalar pronation to supination should occur at approximately the same time in the stance phase, therefore suggesting the possibility of an antagonistic relationship between the two joints through the tibia if these transitions become asynchronous. If pronation continues after knee extension has begun, the tibia will still be internally rotated at the distal end, but an external rotating moment will act at the proximal end of the tibia, creating 'tibial torsional stresses' and abnormal loads on the knee joint.

A further development in running injury research is investigation of intra-participant variability in the coordination of lower extremity joints. This variability was compared in runners with patellofemoral pain syndrome (PFPS) and an asymptomatic control group. It was found that there was less joint coordination variability in patients with PFPS.

Two hypotheses were made regarding this finding. Firstly that the high variability in the asymptomatic group might help attenuate the large impact shocks present during the early stance phase, imparting them to various structures, rather than the same structures being repeatedly loaded as in the low variability group, leading to tissue injury.

The second suggestion was that the decreased variability in the PFPS group could be a result of the PFPS, enabling these individuals to accomplish the task with a minimum of pain. The authors infer that the presence of low phase variability in the lower extremity might be used in the future as an indicator of injury.

Summary

This section has highlighted biomechanical approaches to the identification of aetiological factors that cause overuse injuries in sport and exercise. Few strong links between movements in sport and exercise and specific injuries have been identified, other than the shoulder counter-rotation during the delivery stride of the 'mixed' bowling technique and its association with lower back injuries.

Summary of sports and exercise science

The first part of this chapter has outlined some of the key ways in which sport and exercise science, and in particular the physiology of exercise and

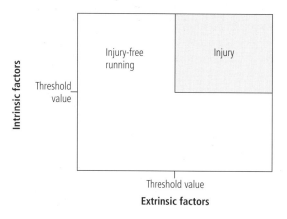

Fig. 3.2 A hypothetical representation of the interaction between intrinsic and extrinsic and potential for injury. Adapted from McCaw (1992).

biomechanics, aid our understanding of factors that underpin performance. Increasingly, scientist, medical practitioner, athlete and coach work together as a team, and this teamwork is essential if the athlete is to be successful during his or her career, and, equally important, later in life when the athlete's competitive days are over.

Sports nutrition

Nutrition significantly influences athletic performance, therefore athletes and their support teams need to understand how to tailor food and fluid intakes to individual requirements, and how to fit refuelling into busy lifestyles.

Key challenges of sports nutrition include maximizing glycogen stores, ensuring adequate protein intake for recovery and repair, preventing dehydration, and optimizing daily nutrient and fluid intake to maximize performance during training and competition.

Sports nutrition should be based on a healthy, well-balanced, high-carbohydrate (CHO), low-fat diet, and as such may be very different from typical Western diets. Ideally 50–60% of calories will be from carbohydrate, 10–15% from protein and <35% from fat. Expressing carbohydrate and protein requirements in grams per kilogram of body weight (g/kg body weight) per day, rather than as percentages of total calories, simplifies calculations. When carbohydrate and protein needs are met, remaining calories can be eaten as fat, because most athletes have adequate fat stores to fuel exercise unless they are restricting caloric intake or have disordered eating. Endurance performance is maximized by a high-carbohydrate rather than a high-fat diet.

Athletes most at risk of nutritional deficiencies are those involved in weight category sports (e.g. judo players and boxers in lightweight categories), or those where physical appearance or low body weight are important (e.g. gymnasts, endurance runners, triathletes).

The information provided here is not designed to replace expert advice from sports scientists and dieticians. However, many doctors and physiotherapists working with non-elite athletes do not have access to such expertise, so they need to know how to identify when food and fluid intakes are inadequate or inappropriate, and how to provide day-to-day refuelling advice.

Fuel for exercise

During exercise, mainly fat and carbohydrate are used as fuel to produce ATP for muscle contraction. At rest, 80–90% of energy comes from fat oxidation, but as exercise intensity increases, increasing amounts are derived from carbohydrate. Utilization of fat by exercising muscles is highest during moderate intensity exercise (around 65% V_{O_2}max), with a progressive shift to carbohydrate at higher intensity, partly because energy is required faster than it can be produced by fat oxidation. Highly trained endurance athletes have increased fat-burning ability, with glycogen-sparing effects. Glycogen stores are limited to around 2000 kcal in males, providing for 60–90 minutes of high-intensity aerobic exercise.

Calculating total calorie needs

If body weight is stable, then energy intake balances energy expenditure. Daily energy requirements can be estimated from the basal metabolic rate (BMR) and level of physical activity. Formulae to allow estimation of daily energy requirements are provided in Table 3.2.

Table 3.2 Calculation of daily energy requirements

Calculation of basic metabolic rate (BMR)		
Age	Males	Females
10–17	$17.5 \times W + 651$	$12.2 \times W + 746$
18–29	$15.3 \times W + 679$	$14.7 \times W + 496$
30–59	$11.6 \times W + 879$	$8.7 \times W + 829$

Calculation of daily energy requirements in kcal		
Activity level	Males	Females
Light	$1.55 \times BMR$	$1.56 \times BMR$
Moderate	$1.78 \times BMR$	$1.64 \times BMR$
Heavy	$2.10 \times BMR$	$1.82 \times BMR$

W = body weight in kilograms.
From FAO/WHO/UNO report 1985.

Completion of a 3–5-day food and fluid intake diary allows estimation of caloric intakes using computer software or food tables. This can be compared with predicted requirements. Unless food is weighed, estimation of portion sizes may be inaccurate.

Carbohydrates

Achieving optimal carbohydrate intake is difficult; therefore athletes need education and encouragement to meet their requirements. Because carbohydrates form such an important part of the athlete's diet, they should be cheap, appealing, suit the individual's taste, provide a variety of flavours, be easy to prepare, carry and eat, and be low in fibre and bulk. Nutrient-dense foods with high carbohydrate content, which also contain protein, vitamins and minerals, are ideal. High glycaemic index (GI) foods, glucose, sucrose and maltodextrins provide readily available carbohydrate to maintain blood glucose levels and rapidly replenish glycogen stores, so are useful during and immediately after exercise. Fructose should be restricted to use post-exercise as it may cause gastrointestinal distress. Lower GI foods induce less marked glucose swings, and lower insulin levels, so are useful at other times.

Calculation of daily carbohydrate requirement

The formula in Table 3.3 can be used to calculate average daily carbohydrate requirements against which to monitor intake. Most athletes underesti-mate their requirements, and without careful planning fail to eat sufficient carbohydrate.

Total carbohydrate requirement should be shared out between three meals, two to three snacks, sports drinks/gels/bars, and post-exercise intake each day. Fifty-gram carbohydrate portions of common foods are shown in Box 3.1. Prepackaged foods have the carbohydrate content on the packet.

A pre-exercise meal (2–4 hours before exercise) containing 1–4 g/kg body weight of carbohydrate optimizes glycogen stores. During high-intensity exercise lasting >60–90 minutes, glycogen stores will be depleted. Some 30–60 g (0.5–1 g/kg body weight) of a high GI carbohydrate per hour during exercise helps maintain blood glucose, spare glycogen stores, and prolong exercise time. Hypotonic or isotonic sports drinks are usually well tolerated during exercise, and contain 5–8% carbohydrate (50–80 g of carbohydrate per litre of reconstituted drink).

Glycogen storage occurs more rapidly during the 2 hours post-exercise. For rapid replenishment, 1 g/kg body weight of a high GI carbohydrate should be consumed in the first 30 minutes post-exercise, followed by 50 g of carbohydrate 2-hourly until the next meal, aiming for 9–10 g/kg body weight over 24 hours.

Sports drinks and gels are convenient, portable and easy to consume, and deliver readily utilized

Table 3.3 Carbohydrate requirements based on daily activity levels

Daily exercise/training	Recommended daily carbohydrate intake to maintain glycogen stores (g/kg body weight/day)
Light (<1 hour)	4–5
Moderate (1–2 hours)	6–7
Heavy (>3 hours)	8–10

Daily carbohydrate requirement (g) = Body weight (kg) multiplied by recommended carbohydrate intake.

Box 3.1 Foods containing 50 g of carbohydrate

1 large bowl cornflakes
2 Shredded Wheat or 3–4 Weetabix
2 bowls of porridge
2 pints of milk
8 tablespoons cooked pasta shapes or 4 tablespoons cooked rice
1 medium baked potato, 5 scoops mashed potato or 5 medium-sized boiled potatoes
4 packets of crisps (3 if low fat)
3–4 slices bread, 1 bagel or 2 rolls
3 slices fruit loaf or Swiss roll
5 digestive biscuits or fig rolls or 6 Jaffa cakes
6 oatcakes, 10 rice cakes or crackers
4 apples, 4 oranges, 3 pears, 2 large bananas, or 60 grapes
7 dates, 5 figs, 20 dried apricots or 3 tablespoons raisins
9 teaspoons jam/honey or 12 teaspoons sugar

carbohydrate and fluid before, during and immediately after exercise, when other food may be poorly tolerated. However, they are no substitute for normal foods, and athletes need guidance on their use.

Protein

Some amino acids are oxidized as fuel, (branched chain amino acids and glutamate, aspartate and asparagine) and all are needed for growth and repair. When carbohydrate intake is adequate, protein provides less than 10% of energy during exercise.

There is no consensus on whether exercise increases protein requirements, although most argue that modestly increased intakes are beneficial in those undertaking regular, strenuous exercise, as shown in Table 3.4. Lower amounts may suffice in females, but there have been few studies. These intakes should be easy to meet from a normal diet (see Table 3.5) and there is no evidence for benefit from protein or amino acid supplements. Athletes should understand that excess protein not required for fuel, repair or renewal will be metabolized and stored as fat.

Animal protein (dairy produce, meat and eggs) contains all the essential amino acids, whereas vegetable protein is deficient in some essential amino acids. Therefore, a combination of vegetable proteins must be consumed to ensure supply of all essential amino acids. Inadequate protein intake may occur in vegetarians, adolescents, pregnant women, 'faddy' eaters, and those restricting food intake to maintain low body weight.

Table 3.4 Calculation of daily protein requirements

Type of exercise	Protein intake recommended (g/kg body weight/day)
Non-athlete	0.8
Strength athlete	1.7–1.8
Endurance athlete	1.2–1.4

Daily protein requirement (g) = Body weight (kg) multiplied by recommended protein intake.

Hydration

Significant decreases in performance can occur with as little as 1–2% dehydration, and sweat losses >1 L/h may occur when exercising on hot days. Rehydration with 600–1200 mL/h of isotonic sports drinks during exercise minimizes dehydration and provides some carbohydrate. Isotonic fluids are well-absorbed during exercise, with absorption best from a relatively full stomach. Athletes need to practise drinking during training to improve tolerance.

Table 3.5 Foods containing 10 g or 20 g of protein

Food	20 g animal protein	Food	10 g vegetable protein
Beef, lamb, pork	75 g/2 slices	Cereal	2 bowls cornflakes, 3 bowls of rice crispies, 7 Weetabix
Turkey, chicken	75 g/1 breast	Bread	4 large slices
Fish	100 g, small fillet	Pasta	8 tablespooons cooked
Salmon/tuna	1 small tin	Rice	12 tablespoons cooked
Fish fingers	6	Biscuits	7 digestive, 6–8 other types
Prawns	2 tablespoons	Nuts	50 g, medium packet
Milk	1 pint	Seeds	50 g, 4 tablespoons
Low-fat yoghurt	3 cartons	Soya milk	350 mL, 2/3 pint
Eggs	3 medium	Baked beans	4 tablespoons
Cheddar cheese	75 g, 2 matchbox size pieces	Kidney beans, lentils	5 tablespoons
Cottage cheese	4 tablespoons	Peanut butter	Thickly spread, 2 slices

From McCance RA, Widdowson EM. *The Composition of Foods*. London, Royal Society of Chemistry, 1991.

Sports drinks contain small amounts of sodium, and this, combined with normal dietary salt intake, is usually adequate to replace losses. If sweat losses are very high, small amounts of rehydration fluid (e.g. Dioralyte) containing higher sodium contents may be useful to prevent hyponatraemia. Salt tablets are not required.

Hydration status can be assessed by examining urine colour or specific gravity, estimating fluid losses by weighing pre- and post-exercise, or by bioimpedance. If weighing, a 1 kg weight loss represents a 1 L fluid loss. Athletes should aim to replace 1.5–2 times fluid losses to allow for ongoing losses. Thirst is a poor indicator of dehydration, so athletes should drink to a plan, rather than relying on thirst. More concentrated carbohydrate drinks (10% or more) can be used to replace some fluid losses and augment carbohydrate intake from food. Addition of small amounts of protein to post-exercise recovery drinks may benefit muscle recovery, but possibly only if carbohydrate intake is suboptimal.

Alcohol- and caffeine-containing drinks are diuretics and are not recommended for fluid replacement. Alcohol should be avoided with soft tissue injuries, as it is a vasodilator and will increase bruising and combat the benefits of rest, ice, compression and elevation (RICE).

Vitamins and minerals

Exercise increases free radical production, so most agree that increased intake of vitamin C (100–500 mg daily) and other antioxidants is required, but these should be supplied by a diet rich in fruits, vegetables, seeds and nuts where possible, rather than by supplements. B vitamins are important for respiratory and neuromuscular functioning, and higher levels of B vitamins may be beneficial in athletes.

Iron losses may be greater in athletes, and iron deficiency is common in females and those on restricted diets. It is hypothesized that low iron stores may affect performance even with normal haemoglobin. Recommended intakes are 7–17 mg/day for male athletes and nonmenstruating females, and 16–23 mg/day for endurance female athletes. These may be hard to achieve, but increased absorption occurs in deficiency states. Nonhaem iron in supple-

ments and vegetables is absorbed better when taken with a source of vitamin C, such as orange juice. Up to 90% of athletes have inadequate zinc intakes, and absorption is decreased by dietary phytates, phosphates, iron and copper. Adequate levels of copper, chromium and selenium are also important. Ideally requirements should be met from the diet rather than supplements, and there is no evidence that supplements in those without deficiencies have any ergogenic effect.

A summary of nutrition advice for competitive athletes is shown in Box 3.2.

Box 3.2 Optimizing nutrition and hydration for competition

- Optimize nutrition during training
- Pre-competition, ensure optimal hydration and replenishment of glycogen stores
  Taper exercise by 50% for a few days pre-competition if possible
  Ensure 8–10 g/kg body weight/day carbohydrate intake for 3 days
  Eat a light, high-carbohydrate meal 2–3 hours or a full meal 4 hours before competition
- Maintain glycogen stores and hydration during endurance events
  Carry sports drinks, gels, bars and snacks if not provided at event
  Begin replacing fluid and carbohydrate early
  Aim for 30–60 g (0.5–1 g/kg body weight) carbohydrate intake per hour
  Replace 80% fluid losses during competition
  Aim for 500–1000 mL isotonic sports drink per hour (in practice only 500–600ml is feasible)
  Keep stomach full to optimize absorption
- Post-competition, rehydrate and replenish glycogen stores rapidly
  Weigh and replace 1.5–2 times predicted fluid losses
  Ensure high GI carbohydrate snacks and drinks available
  Consume 1 g/kg body weight high GI carbohydrates within 30 minutes
  Consume 50–100 g carbohydrate every 2 hours until the first meal
  Aim for 8–10 g/kg body weight carbohydrate in 24 hours
- Always practise nutrition and hydration strategies in training

Ergogenic aids

Ergogenic aids are substances that help increase work output. There is little evidence for the ergogenic potential of legal substances/techniques in endurance exercise apart from appropriate training, maintenance of hydration and glycogen stores, and possibly supplementation with creatine or caffeine.

Some believe that increasing branched chain amino acid intake delays the onset of central fatigue, and that glutamine supplements (5 g single dose after exhaustive exercise) improve immune function, reducing the risk of respiratory infection.

Creatine

Creatine supplements increase muscle creatine phosphate levels, speed recovery from intermittent high-intensity exercise and enhance muscle strength and anaerobic power. Creatine may be most useful in vegetarians who have lower creatine levels. The usual loading regime is 5 g four times daily for 5 days followed by 2 g maintenance daily for 6–8 weeks. Taking creatine with glucose (1 g/kg body weight/day) may produce greater increases in muscle creatine than when taken alone. Fluid retention, weight gain and muscle cramps are all side effects that may occur, with renal impairment having also been reported.

Caffeine

Caffeine increases lipolysis, enhances fatty acid oxidation and may spare glycogen stores, possibly enhancing endurance performance.

Weight category sports

Athletes need to be realistic when choosing a weight category for competition, and should stay within 1–2 kg of this weight during training. Reducing salt consumption for 7 days before weigh-in, and eating a low-residue diet for the final 24 hours should ensure they 'make weight' safely. Saunas and laxatives are illegal, and dehydration and starvation should be avoided. To optimize performance, and reduce injury risk, rehydration and replenishment of glycogen stores should be a priority between weigh-in and competition.

4 Sports injuries of the shoulder

Anatomy

The shoulder comprises four separate joints: the glenohumeral joint, the scapulothoracic joint, the acromioclavicular joint and the sternoclavicular joint (Fig. 4.1). It is a joint designed to maximize the functional efficiency of our hands and therefore has an extraordinary range of movement, unfortunately at the cost of joint stability.

Sternoclavicular joint

This small saddle joint (Fig. 4.1) is the only bone-to-bone connection between the upper limb and the trunk. Despite this unique role, structural stability has been compromised to facilitate a significant range of movement. A fibrocartilaginous disc pro-

vides stability and shock absorption. A number of ligaments provide additional static stability.

Acromioclavicular joint (ACJ)

This is a plane joint, providing a limited amount of gliding and rotation between the clavicle and scapula (Fig. 4.1). Joint stability is almost entirely dependent on ligamentous support, primarily the superior acromioclavicular and coracoclavicular (conoid and trapezoid) ligaments.

Glenohumeral joint

This multiaxial ball joint is the most freely mobile joint of the body (Fig. 4.1). Accordingly, a complex interaction exists between static and dynamic

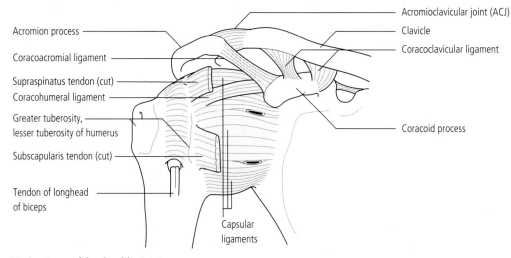

Acromion process

Coracoacromial ligament

Supraspinatus tendon (cut)

Coracohumeral ligament

Greater tuberosity,
lesser tuberosity of humerus

Subscapularis tendon (cut)

Tendon of longhead
of biceps

Capsular
ligaments

Acromioclavicular joint (ACJ)

Clavicle

Coracoclavicular ligament

Coracoid process

Fig. 4.1 Anatomy of the shoulder joint.

stabilizers to provide support. Static stability is provided by the glenoid labrum, a fibrocartilaginous rim that increases the available contact area of the glenoid by about 70%, and the capsule with its intrinsic ligaments, the glenohumeral ligaments. The labrum is the primary attachment site for the shoulder capsule and glenohumeral ligaments. At its superior aspect it is also the attachment site for the long head of biceps tendon. Thus the labrum is crucial to glenohumeral stability by extending the glenoid cavity and by providing anchorage for both static and dynamic stabilizers of the glenohumeral joint.

Dynamic support is provided by the rotator cuff and long head of biceps. The rotator cuff comprises the four tendons of interrelated muscles, which all take origin from the scapula, the supraspinatus, infraspinatus, teres minor and subscapularis.

Scapulothoracic joint

The scapula, only attached to the skeleton at the acromioclavicular joint, glides around the chest wall (Fig. 4.1). Scapula control is vital to upper limb function as it provides a mobile platform from which the upper limb can operate. This control is dependent on complex interactions between coupled agonist and antagonist muscles including levator scapulae, rhomboids, serratus anterior, trapezius and the pectorals.

The shoulder joint complex

Assessment of the painful shoulder is complicated by the polyarticular nature of shoulder movement and the tendency for pain to refer to the shoulder. It is further complicated by the overlap between different pathologies, for example rotator cuff tendinopathy, capsular inflammation and instability. Many pathologies have both acute and chronic presentations, and so in categorizing these injuries it is more reasonable to look at each anatomical region.

Impingement

Often described as a pathological entity, impingement is a symptom not a diagnosis, with the athlete complaining of 'pain with overhead activity'. It can be a consequence of rotator cuff pathology (see below), as the swollen tissues, usually supraspina-

tus, are compressed within the subacromial space by the acromion and coracoacromial ligament.

Conversely it can be the cause of rotator cuff damage, the impingement occurring secondarily to factors such as glenohumeral instability, biomechanical abnormalities that may relate to poor technique or muscle imbalances causing altered scapulothoracic coordination, and anatomical factors such as acromion anomalies or subacromial osteophytes.

Pain is most significant in the abducted and internally rotated position, occurring in activities such as freestyle swimming or during the follow-through of the throwing action.

Impingement tests

These are tests that are used to produce the clinical symptomatology of impingement, the findings then being further refined to achieve a diagnosis:
- Painful arc – pain noted during the abduction phase, usually commencing at around 90°.
- Pain with overpressure of the adducted/internally rotated shoulder, flexed to 90° (empty can sign).
- Pain reproduction generated by forward flexion and internal rotation of the abducted shoulder (Hawkins sign).

The management of impingement is therefore multifactorial, the aim being to correct any causative factors and to treat the underlying pathology.

Injuries of the shoulder joint complex

Injuries may be separated into the following categories:
1 Musculotendinous injuries (rotator cuff, biceps, pectoral).
2 Glenohumeral joint pathology (adhesive capsulitis, labral injuries, glenohumeral instability and dislocation).
3 Other joint and bony injuries (ACJ, clavicular, sternoclavicular).

Musculotendinous injuries

The rotator cuff
Presentation
Rotator cuff injuries may present acutely or chronically depending on the underlying causation and pathology.

The following conditions may occur within the rotator cuff:

- acute tendinitis;
- musculotendinous tear;
- tendinopathy.

The throwing action requires the coordinated firing of the four rotator cuff muscles, in unison with a stable scapulothoracic joint. During the follow-through phase, the subscapularis is working concentrically to internally rotate the arm, while the supraspinatus, infraspinatus and teres minor are working eccentrically to decelerate the arm. This repetitive eccentric activity can lead to overload and as a consequence 'repetitive microtrauma'.

This can present acutely as rotator cuff tendonitis (usually supraspinatus), with recurrent episodes suggesting the possibility of an underlying tendinopathy. Sudden trauma, for instance following a dislocation or fall – the latter being a particularly common presentation in the older athlete in sports such as rugby – may indicate a rotator cuff tear.

Presenting symptoms are typically of poorly localized pain in the shoulder region, often with a referral into the upper arm and sometimes down the forearm, even into the hand. This can cause confusion when trying to differentiate this presentation from pain associated with cervical spine pathology. Symptoms described are usually those of the classical painful arc, with discomfort during overhead activity and often exacerbated by lying on the affected side.

Diagnosis
The history has usually given a good indication as to the acute, chronic or traumatic nature of the underlying pathology. Examination findings vary; however, they usually include positive impingement tests (described above), with associated weakness on resisted testing of the involved portions of the rotator cuff.

Wasting is occasionally present, most often following a partial or full-thickness tear. Research has shown that it is difficult to reliably report which element of the rotator cuff is responsible for underlying symptoms based on palpation, which is therefore often unhelpful, although the shoulder will usually present with generalized tenderness.

Ultrasound is one of the most useful and least invasive forms of investigation used to demonstrate rotator cuff pathology. Impingement may be visualized dynamically, with tendinopathy, partial or full-thickness tears and associated subacromial bursitis being clearly visible to the experienced operator.

Magnetic resonance imaging (MRI) is also of use in this situation; however, a significant proportion of labral and rotator cuff pathology is missed due to the static nature of this form of investigation.

Management
Initial management should include the control of pain, relative rest and appropriate use of nonsteroidal anti-inflammatory drugs (NSAIDs).

In the case of impingement associated with more minor rotator cuff pathology such as tendonitis with possible associated subacromial bursitis, range of motion is gradually restored, exercises being progressed initially through a painless range. Gaining scapular control is an important part of the rehabilitation process, with a progression to more sports-specific exercises commencing when initial phases have been successfully completed. At this stage a review of technique and equipment should also be undertaken.

Persistent tendonitis with or without subacromial bursitis may respond to corticosteroid injection into the subacromial space.

In nonresponsive cases, associated pathology such as a cuff tear, tendinosis or labral pathology, should be considered even when accompanied by normal radiology, and diagnostic arthroscopy may be indicated.

Acute rotator cuff tears confirmed clinically and radiologically in young otherwise healthy patients, require surgical repair. This is now usually performed arthroscopically. Subacromial decompression is frequently performed at the same time.

Older patients tend to present with chronic tears of a degenerate rotator cuff. Their management reflects the functional limitations and expectations of the patient, and the size and depth of the tear. Small tears are frequently managed conservatively. Large tears may be repairable; however, if the rotator cuff is degenerate it may be preferable to address the patient's pain by performing subacromial decompression.

Biceps tendon rupture
Most ruptures involve the proximal long head of biceps and produce the classical 'Popeye' deformity. Isolated rupture is unusual and it frequently reflects

coincident impingement and degeneration, thus it is usually seen in older athletes. Management is usually conservative.

Rupture in younger individuals may be seen in weightlifters and has been linked to the use of anabolic steroids. Strong-man competitors may rupture their distal biceps tendon, resulting in weakened elbow supination and flexion, and consideration should therefore be given to surgical repair.

Pectoralis major rupture
Presentation
This is a relatively unusual injury but one that requires careful consideration because of the important role of the pectoralis major. Rupture may be partial or complete and is usually a result of a sudden force on an actively contracting muscle, for example weightlifting or breaking a fall while climbing. Occasionally rupture may occur following a direct blow. Injury to the distal insertion, distal musculotendinous junction or muscle belly are most likely.

Diagnosis
In the acute stages swelling and bruising are obvious and these may obscure the classical sign of a distal tear, loss of the anterior axillary fold. Resisted contraction, if tolerated, will accentuate the deformity. Chronic tears will present with obvious deformity and asymmetry (unless of course there are bilateral tears).

Investigation comprises ultrasound, which will readily establish the site of a tear; however, it may not be possible to differentiate partial from complete tears and consequently MRI may be required.

Management
Partial tears may be managed conservatively, and recovery is likely to take 6–8 weeks. Complete tears in those whose sport requires upper limb strength are best treated with surgical repair.

Glenohumeral joint pathology

Adhesive capsulitis ('frozen shoulder')
Presentation
The aetiology is unknown, but this condition seems to be precipitated by minor episodes of trauma in some patients.

Clinical presentation is usually one of painful restriction of active and passive movement of the glenohumeral joint. Patients' symptoms frequently evolve through an initial stage of pain, followed by stiffness and finally recovery. Full recovery may take 2 years or more, although it has been postulated that recovery is proportional to the length of the painful phase.

Diagnosis
Examination in the early stages demonstrates a restriction of external rotation, and early scapular movement during shoulder abduction (i.e. a capsular pattern). This differentiates it from other shoulder pathologies, those associated with impingement presenting with restricted painful internal rotation. Severe pain and global restriction of glenohumeral movement occur as the condition progresses.

Plain X-rays are undertaken to exclude glenohumeral arthropathy. Further investigations are not required.

Management
This is a condition rarely seen in athletes, but when it does occur it does not respond readily to treatment. Aggressive treatment of the painful phase may speed up recovery, with the use of NSAIDs, encouragement of painless range of motion (ROM) exercises, and consideration of hydrodilatation with combined local anaesthetic and corticosteroid.

Labral injury
Presentation
Injury to the glenoid labrum is a frequently missed cause of shoulder pain and loss of function. This largely reflects a failure to recognize the potential for labral injury.

The glenoid labrum is a fibrocartilaginous ring that extends the diameter and depth of the glenoid cavity (Fig. 4.1). Excessive traction may damage the labrum, particularly during activities such as carrying, pitching, swimming or tennis. Compression forces can also produce injury and may occur during a fall on an externally rotated arm.

Pain is often poorly localized and exacerbated by overhead and behind-the-back movements. A history of grinding, popping or catching may be described. Patients may also report an episode of trauma.

Diagnosis

Injury to the labrum is usually accompanied by subtle signs, making diagnosis more difficult and the history more important. Anterosuperior glenohumeral pain is not uncommon. Several diagnostic tests have been reported but these appear to have only modest sensitivity and specificity:

• Anterior slide test
• Empty can test
• Crank test – analogous to the Apley's grind test for meniscal tears.

Testing the shoulder through various resisted ranges of motion, particularly those positions into which the shoulder is placed during competition and training, can be helpful.

Investigation consists of MR arthrography, with normal MRI, as discussed, often not being sufficient to exclude a labral tear.

Labral injuries often become a diagnosis of exclusion, and nonresolving cases of shoulder pain even with accompanying negative radiology should be referred for arthroscopy as the final definitive form of investigation.

Management

As discussed above, SLAP (superior labrum anterior to posterior) lesions are usually only considered once conservative treatment of shoulder pain has failed. Consequently, when such lesions are diagnosed, referral for arthroscopic repair is often indicated. SLAP lesions can, however, be classified according to the involvement of the biceps insertion, and this is said to define those that ultimately require surgery because of the consequent instability (Fig. 4.2).

Glenohumeral instability and dislocation

Instability may be classified in a number of ways including its direction (anterior, posterior, multidirectional) and its cause (traumatic, atraumatic).

Presentation

The glenohumeral joint is the most frequently dislocated joint. Ninety percent of dislocations are anterior, usually resulting from a fall onto an abducted and externally rotated arm (see 'Skiing and snowboarding' in Chapter 16). In the majority, the labrum and attached inferior glenohumeral ligament is disrupted, producing the Bankart lesion. The other

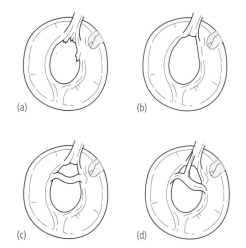

Fig. 4.2 Grading of SLAP lesions. (a) Fraying and degeneration is seen around the labrum. (b) Glenoid labrum and long head of biceps are detached. (c) Labrum is torn away but bicep attachment intact. (d) Labrum and long head of bicep torn and displaced. (NB (b) and (d) are associated with shoulder instability and require repair.)

major pathological sequela of shoulder dislocation is the Hill–Sachs lesion, which is a fracture of the posterolateral humeral head as it becomes impacted on the antero-inferior glenoid rim.

The severity of the injury is usually obvious; however, it is important to ascertain injury mechanism and arm position. The patient usually presents with severe pain and the arm held at the side.

Atraumatic instability presents with a more insidious onset. Sports such as gymnastics, swimming, diving (Fig. 4.3), tennis and throwing field events (e.g. javelin) predominate, as a result of their requirement for an increased range of motion in the glenohumeral joint in association with repeated overhead activity. The complaint may simply be of recurrent shoulder pain caused by irritation of the rotator cuff and capsule; however, in some cases the individual arrives complaining that the arm has 'gone dead' following throwing activities or a particularly vigorous manoeuvre. This is known not surprisingly as 'dead arm syndrome' and is a recognized presenting symptom in cases of anterior instability.

Diagnosis

In the case of dislocation, further inspection reveals that the normal contour of the deltoid and acromion

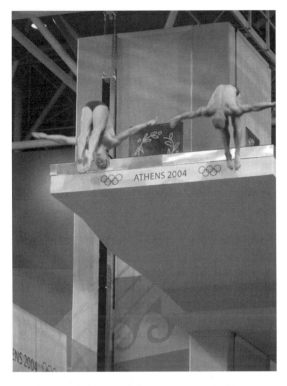

Fig. 4.3 Atraumatic instability may present in divers.

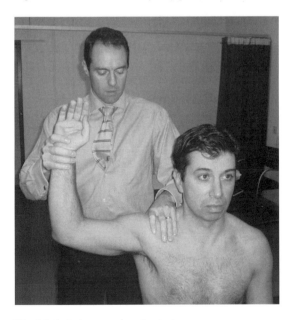

Fig. 4.4 Anterior apprehension test.

is lost. A full neurovascular examination must be performed before any attempt at relocation. Particular attention should be paid to the axillary nerve, although sensory disturbance to the lateral aspect of the shoulder does not appear to be a reliable sign, with resisted testing of the deltoid being a more objective indicator of axillary nerve status.

Functional stability testing is not required in the acute setting; however, it is useful in terms of assessing the stability of a shoulder that has been previously dislocated as an indicator of further management and will obviously help confirm the diagnosis in cases of atraumatic instability.

Anterior stability tests. **Apprehension test** – patient supine or sat and the shoulder abducted and externally rotated (Fig. 4.4).
AP (anteroposterior) translation test – feeling for excessive anterior translation of the humeral head beyond the normal 50% of the width of the glenoid.

Inferior stability tests. **Sulcus sign** – with the patient sat, a sulcus is seen as downward traction is applied to the humerus.

Generalized laxity. Atraumatic shoulder instability may reflect a generalized predisposition to joint laxity, and this should be assessed by examining other joints (wrist, little finger, elbow, knee) for signs of hypermobility (the Beighton criteria).

Investigations. These should consist of true AP, transscapular and axillary view X-rays to confirm the direction of the dislocation and to exclude a fracture.

Management

Uncomplicated anterior dislocation is usually managed with closed reduction, for which a number of techniques are reported. Open reduction is reserved for failed closed reduction, where there is neurovascular injury (either before or after closed reduction) and for fracture dislocations. Neurovascular re-examination must take place after closed reduction. Any change in neurovascular status requires urgent surgical evaluation.

Successful rehabilitation requires adequate time for the anterior glenohumeral ligaments to heal and thus abduction and external rotation must be avoided for at least 6 weeks. Other range of motion exercises are performed early, with a gradual progression over the first 4–6 weeks. A return to sport must not be undertaken until the rehabilitation is complete, with a successful progression through the graduated sports-specific exercises. Even with careful rehabilitation, redislocation is reported in over 60% of active young patients, and therefore for those involved in sport, particularly contact sport, surgical reconstruction is recommended.

Posterior dislocation is rare and usually takes the form of subluxation (often as a manifestation of generalized hypermobility) rather then true dislocation. Anatomical deformity is less obvious and careful attention needs to be paid to X-ray changes so as not to miss the diagnosis. Epileptic seizure or electrocution are two other situations associated with this condition. Labral and bony injury is unusual, with surgical repair not usually being required.

Atraumatic instability is managed conservatively, using a regime of rotator cuff strengthening and scapular stabilizing exercises.

Occasionally this approach is unsuccessful and a surgical procedure is necessary to stabilize the joint. In unilateral instability this approach is often helpful; however, in cases of multidirectional instability the outcomes are not as favourable.

Other joint and bony injuries

Acromioclavicular joint injury
Presentation
Injury to the acromioclavicular joint (ACJ) usually occurs following a direct blow, a fall on the point of the shoulder or a fall onto an outstretched hand. It is most commonly seen in contact sports such as rugby.

Inspection will often note a prominence of the clavicle with palpation demonstrating pain localized to the ACJ, this being a joint that localizes pain well with little or no referral.

Examination reveals shoulder pain produced by movement in all directions, with the adduction stress test (Scarf test) causing particular discomfort.

Management
Injury is usually graded 1, 2 or 3 depending on severity (Table 4.1). Plain X-rays are required to assess the degree of separation and to exclude a fracture.

Clavicular fractures
These fractures are classified according to their location (middle, distal or proximal thirds) and by the amount of angulation, comminution and displacement of the fracture site. The proximal segment is usually drawn superiorly by the sternocleidomastoid muscle. The distal segment drops under the effect of gravity.

Uncomplicated fractures can be treated conservatively with a sling for 6–8 weeks. Moderate displacement might require the use of a figure-of-eight bandage. Failed conservative management, tenting of the skin or neurovascular injury require surgical fixation. Traditionally the last resort, surgeons are increasingly reporting accelerated restoration of function for athletes with mid-clavicular fractures (see 'Further reading').

Traumatic osteolysis
Repetitive trauma may result in osteolysis, which is seen as distal clavicular resorption and cyst formation on X-ray. Patients present with pain. Those at risk include rugby players, ice hockey players and weightlifters.

Table 4.1 Acromioclavicular joint injury

Grade	Examination findings	Management
1	Swelling, tenderness but no deformity	Early mobilization. Activity within limits of pain
2	Ligamentous disruption although coracoclavicular ligaments intact. Swelling, tenderness with some subluxation	Joint protection (sling) to prevent further damage. Mobilization within limits of pain
3	Complete joint disruption with considerable deformity and instability. Pain and swelling	Grade 3 injuries may require surgical repair depending on the extent of trauma/joint disruption and separation

Sternoclavicular injury

Sternoclavicular injuries are less common than ACJ injuries, but can also be divided into grade 1, 2 or 3 sprains. Grade 3 injuries (dislocation) may be further classified as either posterior or anterior, depending on whether the medial clavicle is anterior or posterior to the sternum. Grade 1 and 2 injuries are managed conservatively with a sling for comfort and then progressive range of movement exercises within the limits of pain. Anterior dislocation is managed by closed reduction, best achieved by placing the patient on a rolled towel between the scapulae.

Posterior dislocations are potentially serious because of the close proximity to pulmonary and vascular structures. Open reduction may be required if careful closed reduction is unsuccessful; however, this procedure is not without significant risk and often marks the end of the patient's career in sports such as gymnastics.

Summary

It is questionable that there is a more challenging musculoskeletal problem than a patient with shoulder pain. That said an appreciation of the functional anatomy of the shoulder complex and a realization that shoulder pain may be referred from elsewhere, or may reflect a secondary injury from a primary problem within the kinetic chain, should enable the clinician to reach a differential diagnosis and management plan.

Further reading

Jubel A, Andemahr J, Bergmann H *et al.* Elastic stable intramedullary nailing of midclavicular fractures in athletes. *Br J Sports Med* 2003, **37**(6), 480–3; discussion 484.

5 Sports injuries to the upper limb, hand and wrist

This chapter will deal with injury to the elbow, wrist and hand. Upper arm injuries, such as biceps tendon rupture, have already been dealt with in Chapter 4.

Anatomy of the elbow, forearm and wrist (Fig. 5.1)

The elbow is a compound synovial hinge joint, with articulations between the olecranon of the ulna and the trochlea of the humerus, and the head of the radius with the capitulum of the humerus. There are capsular collateral ligaments providing resistance to varus and valgus strain. The radial head is held in position by the annular ligament, which is a strong band attached mainly to the ulnar notch.

The elbow joint connects with the proximal radio-ulnar joint, the radius pivoting on a static ulna during

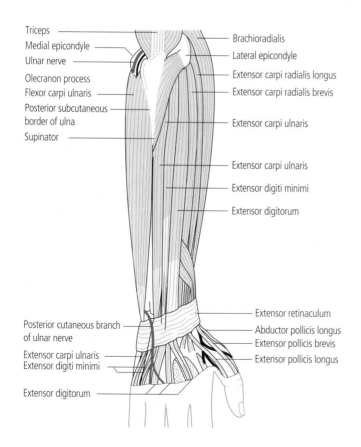

Triceps
Medial epicondyle
Ulnar nerve
Olecranon process
Flexor carpi ulnaris
Posterior subcutaneous border of ulna
Supinator

Brachioradialis
Lateral epicondyle
Extensor carpi radialis longus
Extensor carpi radialis brevis

Extensor carpi ulnaris

Extensor carpi ulnaris
Extensor digiti minimi
Extensor digitorum

Posterior cutaneous branch of ulnar nerve
Extensor carpi ulnaris
Extensor digiti minimi
Extensor digitorum

Extensor retinaculum
Abductor pollicis longus
Extensor pollicis brevis
Extensor pollicis longus

Fig 5.1 Anatomy of the elbow and wrist.

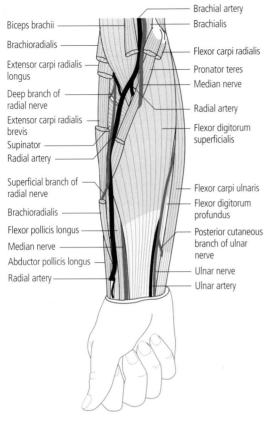
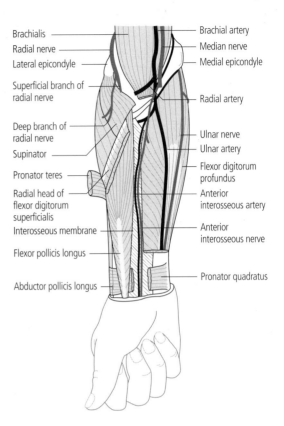

Fig 5.1 (Continued.)

the movements of pronation and supination. The interosseus membrane is a fibrous connection (a syndesmosis) between the medial border of the radius and the lateral border of the ulna, the fibres passing diagonally downwards from radius to ulna. It affords attachment to the deep muscles of the forearm, whilst also transmitting forces from the radius to the ulna when an axial load is applied, for example in a fall onto the hand. The distal radio-ulnar joint is also a pivot joint, allowing the actions of pronation and supination.

Elbow pain

This section will divide the causes of elbow pain into acute and chronic categories, starting with the latter, due to its importance and frequent presentation in sport. The differential diagnosis of upper limb pain should always consider the possibility of referred pain from the cervical spine.

Chronic elbow injuries

Flexor and extensor tendinosis (medial and lateral epicondylosis)

The long flexors and extensors of the wrist and hand originate from relatively small attachments on the medial and lateral side of the elbow, the epicondyles.

Extensor tendinosis (tennis elbow)

Presentation

Also a frequent occurrence in the nonsporting population, it is usually the racket sports player who presents with this problem, the underlying mechanism being that of repeated wrist extension. However, although this condition has acquired the name 'tennis elbow', it is not uncommon in golfers. The player will complain of pain on activity, arising either acutely or progressively worsening over a period of time, with the older player, usually 35 years and upwards, being more commonly affected.

Diagnosis

Resisting wrist extension will classically reproduce symptoms, with discomfort also being experienced on stretching the musculo-tendinous junction by fully flexing and pronating the wrist with elbow extension. Palpation will reveal tenderness just distal to the epicondyle, where the tendon of extensor carpi radialis brevis (ECRB) is located, the pathology appearing to be a tendinotic change within this structure. There is much debate as to the underlying cause of the tendinosis; however, the combination of repeated microtrauma and inadequate rehabilitation appears to be responsible.

Investigation is not usually necessary as this is a clinical diagnosis; however, ultrasound will support the diagnosis. Further investigation is only required when the diagnosis is unclear.

Management

Many presentations will be an acute on chronic exacerbation of the condition and so the usual approaches aimed at reducing any acute inflammation and maintaining range of motion are initially followed.

Once the acute symptoms have settled, soft tissue therapy is introduced followed by a rehabilitation programme, which should involve progressive loading of the structure, eventually incorporating eccentric exercises.

Bracing, in the form of an epicondylar clasp, can be used both in the rehabilitation process or to prevent a recurrence. This appears to work by changing the angle of 'pull' of the tendon at its origin.

Additional factors such as inappropriate technique and equipment may be contributory and should be assessed. Attempts to generate power and spin by using excessive amounts of 'wrist' in the serve or forehand are often implicated, as is a faulty backhand technique.

Racket grip size, weight and string tension can all be aggravating factors, and although temporary relief may be obtained with the treatments outlined, the problem will return unless these factors are addressed in full.

Corticosteroid injection may be considered in those that fail to respond, although this should only be undertaken alongside an ongoing rehabilitation programme, because when undertaken in isolation this treatment tends to produce only temporary reso-

lution of symptoms. Autologous blood injection is at present undergoing review as a possible treatment.

Intractable cases sometimes progress to surgery, with the procedure involving debridement of the ECRB tendon and surgical tenotomy.

Flexor tendinosis (golfer's elbow)

This condition occurs both in golfers and those participating in racket sports, with the pathology occurring at the common flexor origin. Presentation occurs in a similar manner to that described in extensor tendinosis, with pain on activity and localized tenderness.

Examination will also demonstrate discomfort on resisted wrist flexion.

Management guidelines are similar to those described above, with the golf swing requiring attention, as again does the 'wristy' topspin forehand.

Thrower's elbow

Presentation

During throwing, the cocking and acceleration phases of the action impart significant stresses on the elbow joint. Valgus overload compresses the lateral side of the joint (radio-humeral area), whilst tensioning the medial side (ulno-humeral area). This is a common occurrence in throwers (e.g. javelin throwers or baseball pitchers) and may present either acutely or chronically, the different pathologies being described below.

Diagnosis

The main pathology involves injury to the medial collateral ligament, which as mentioned can present as an acute strain or following repeated microtrauma, the latter leading to chronic ligamentous laxity, with scarring and calcification.

Repeated loading in the presence of ligamentous damage and joint laxity can then result in joint damage, loose body formation and occasionally ulnar neuritis.

In young baseball pitchers, this is the basis of 'little leaguer's elbow', which comprises a traction apophysitis, combined with osteochondritis dissecans (OCD) of the capitellum and loose body formation (occurring in the older child, e.g. 13–16 years).

Panner's disease is one of osteochondroses occurring in the younger population (7–12 years) and must be considered here. It is due to a disruption of the capitellar ossification centre, and the important differentiation from OCD is made on the basis of age and imaging.

Examination may demonstrate a joint effusion, best seen from behind, with generalized tenderness, and pain on both flexion and extension. Locking may occur due to associated loose bodies.

Lateral X-ray views may reveal a shadow just posterior to the olecranon fossa, the 'fat pad sign', indicating the presence of an effusion. In OCD, subchondral bony involvement may be demonstrated.

Magnetic resonance imaging (MRI) will reveal the true extent of the damage, clearly defining the soft tissue pathology and intra-articular damage. A computed tomography (CT) scan may then be required if advanced OCD is demonstrated and bony involvement is suspected.

Management
In the early stages of these conditions, management follows a similar pattern to that of epicondylosis. Panner's disease is always managed conservatively, whereas the more advanced cases of OCD or those involving loose bodies may require surgical intervention.

In severe intractable cases associated with excessive joint laxity, ligamentous reconstruction is sometimes undertaken; however, this is very much a last resort.

A chronically scarred ligament is also prone to rupture if overloaded with an excessive valgus force.

Nerve entrapment syndromes
Posterior interosseous nerve
The posterior interosseus nerve runs through the supinator muscle, where it may become entrapped, causing pain that at first glance may be indistinguishable from that of extensor tendinosis. However, further examination will reveal that the focus of pain is below the epicondyle itself.

Ulnar nerve
The ulnar nerve runs in its groove 1 cm posterior to the epicondyle, and may become involved in the inflammatory process, with the possibility of subsequent scarring. Symptoms and signs of ulnar nerve involvement are present, with paraesthesiae radiating into the ring finger and little finger. Tenderness

is present at or just distal to the epicondyle and over the nerve in the cubital fossa, with Tinel's test also being positive.

Management
Nerve conduction studies may be necessary to confirm the diagnosis, and the management of both conditions then involves the use of local soft tissue therapy and neural stretches. Intractable cases of ulnar nerve compression may require surgical intervention, consisting of nerve transfer, with the nerve being moved around the epicondyle, to lie deep to the flexor muscles.

Acute elbow injuries

Posterior elbow dislocation
Presentation
Posterior elbow dislocation mainly occurs between the ages of 5 and 25 years, and accounts for 20% of all dislocations. During a fall, the natural carrying angle allows for an abduction force to be applied to the joint, aiding the dislocation force. As with supracondylar fractures, there is a risk of vascular impairment following this injury, and a careful assessment of the peripheral vascular status should be carried out. If there is vascular compromise, immediate reduction should be attempted. Associated fractures of the coronoid process anteriorly, or of the radial head, are not uncommon.

Diagnosis
Examination reveals a palpable prominence of the olecranon process posteriorly. The normal relationship between it and the epicondyles is lost (unlike supracondylar fracture). Urgent review of the neurovascular status is vital. Plain lateral X-ray will demonstrate the deformity, and any associated fractures.

Management
Reduction can often be undertaken immediately, with traction being applied to the forearm, which is held at 30–45°. Vascular status should be repeatedly checked. Myositis ossifans may be a delayed complication of this injury. Indomethacin, if not contraindicated, appears to decrease the likelihood of this occurring.

Olecranon bursitis

This is a condition that usually occurs following a fall onto a hard surface. Basketball and volleyball players therefore predominate. There is usually a significant effusion within the bursa, and the routine of rest, ice and compression is followed acutely. Some cases will fail to resolve and so aspiration with corticosteroid injection is undertaken under sterile conditions, so as to prevent the introduction of infection. Intractable cases occasionally proceed to surgical resection.

Triceps tendinitis/rupture

This condition is not common, but is seen in weight-lifters and in some field event competitors, such as shot-putters.

The usual management regime is followed in line with the treatment of any acute musculotendinous injury.

Very occasionally, acute rupture of the triceps tendon occurs following a fall. Surgical repair is indicated.

The **biceps tendon** has been mentioned previously in relation to its ruptured long head in the shoulder; however, this muscle can also rupture at its insertion and likewise requires acute repair.

Avulsion of the medial epicondyle

The medial epicondyle is the last epiphysis to unite with the shaft of the humerus. It does so in the 20th year. Injury occurs following forced wrist extension (e.g. martial arts), with the epicondyle becoming avulsed from the shaft of the humerus.

Examination reveals pain locally and on forced wrist dorsiflexion, with the avulsion being demonstrated on plain X-rays.

Management involves open reduction and internal fixation (ORIF) and with adequate rehabilitation, the patient should recover fully.

Forearm injuries

Radial and ulnar fractures

Fractures of the forearm occur following a direct blow or a fall. The following presentations are seen.

Fractures of both forearm bones

These occur following local trauma, with the action of the muscle groups on each of the bones causing deformities, often making reduction difficult.

Examination findings are of pain, swelling and deformity. Vascular status must be checked. Plain X-ray will confirm the extent of the injury.

Open reduction and internal fixation is the treatment of choice for many, as the continued muscular action on the fractured bones means that manipulation and immobilization in a cast will not maintain position.

Fractures of single forearm bones

With single bone fractures, there is often an associated dislocation. For this reason, X-rays of the whole forearm, including both radio-ulnar joints, should be carried out. (N.B. an ulnar fracture with radial head dislocation is a Monteggia fracture; a radial fracture with inferior radio-ulnar joint subluxation is a Galeazzi fracture.)

On examination in the case of the Monteggia fracture, the ulnar deformity is obvious; however, if there is major swelling the radial head injury may be obscured. Palpation will elicit pain at this site. The radial nerve may be involved and should be assessed.

Following a Galeazzi fracture the distal ulnar deformity is easily seen, with pain and swelling associated with the fracture site. The ulnar nerve may be involved and should be assessed. Plain X-rays will again confirm the injury.

Management in the adult usually consists of open reduction and fixation, as the integrated mechanics of the forearm require the length of the fractured bone to be restored. A late complication can occur known as 'night stick injury' (so called because of the ulnar fractures sustained in beatings during arrests in the USA), when a block to extension occurs as a result of shortening of the healed ulna, as the radial head is forced upwards into the capitulum.

Compartment syndrome

This condition may occur acutely following the above mentioned traumatic injuries or as a chronic condition associated with activities such as windsurfing or canoeing (Fig. 5.2). Compartment pressure testing will confirm the diagnosis, with most cases then settling conservatively; surgical decompression is occasionally required.

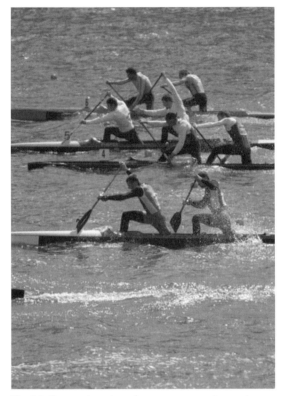

Fig. 5.2 Compartment syndrome may occur in sports such as canoeing.

Stress fractures

Any sport that involves excessive upper limb use may result in the production of a stress fracture. Racket sports and activities such as rowing therefore predominate.

However, stress fractures of the forearm are relatively uncommon compared with the frequency of this condition in the leg, for instance.

The wrist joint

The wrist joint, or radiocarpal joint, is formed between the distal end of the radius and articular disc, and the proximal carpal bones. It is a biaxial/ellipsoid synovial joint. Although it would appear that the distal end of the ulna articulates with the medial proximal carpus (lunate and triquetral), the articular disc intercedes between the two. The disc is fibrocartilaginous, and is attached to the medial side of the radius and the lateral border of the ulnar styloid.

Collateral as well as anterior and posterior ligaments support the radiocarpal joint.

There are two rows of carpal bones, with the proximal row constituting the distal part of the radiocarpal joint, whilst both rows constitute the intercarpal joints. The movements at the radiocarpal and intercarpal joints are interlinked, and should be considered together. They are flexion and extension (with similar ranges of approximately 85°), adduction (approximately 45°) and abduction (approximately 15°). There are intercarpal ligamentous connections, as well as collateral ligament support. The metacarpal bones articulate with the distal row of the carpal bones and the proximal phalanges. There are three phalanges in each finger and two in the thumb, with all joints being synovial. The intercarpal ligaments lie just below the level of the metacarpophalangeal joints (MCPs), with the collateral ligaments being associated with the interphalangeal joints (IPJs) and the MCPs.

The most common types of wrist injury in the athlete are traumatic, although chronic and overuse injuries cause considerable morbidity. The acute injuries will therefore be discussed first. Combat sports, gymnastics, diving (Fig. 5.3), snowboarding and racket sports all produce injuries, with golf also producing frequent presentations – in one survey (undertaken at the European Open in Porthcawl, 2002) more than half of professional golfers recounted some history of wrist injury.

Acute wrist injuries

Distal radial and ulnar fractures

Invariably these are sustained when falling awkwardly. The fracture may involve the joint(s). Pain, swelling and deformity are noted on examination, with plain X-ray confirming the diagnosis.

Management consists of manipulation and cast immobilization.

Scaphoid fracture

Fracture is usually sustained following a fall onto an outstretched hand. Examination classically reveals tenderness on palpation within the anatomical snuff box, with discomfort also elicited when pressure is applied over the scaphoid tubercle.

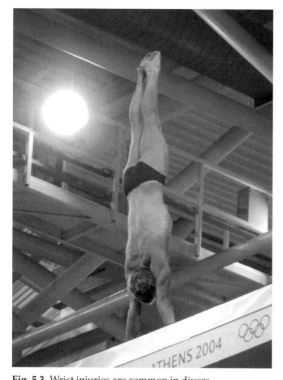

Fig. 5.3 Wrist injuries are common in divers.

Plain X-rays often show no abnormality in the acute phase. If the index of suspicion is high, then isotope bone scan or CT scan will help confirm the diagnosis. However, an MRI scan will give a positive result within six hours of injury and may become the norm as its availability increases. A plain X-ray 7–10 days after the injury would also demonstrate the healing fracture.

Early diagnosis and management is essential, with delay sometimes leading to nonunion and avascular necrosis. Immobilization in a plaster of Paris (POP) is therefore undertaken if there is any suspicion of a fracture, and this continues for a minimum of 8 weeks (12 weeks being the median time to union), as those removed from cast at 6 weeks demonstrate an increased incidence of nonunion. Fractures demonstrating greater than 2 mm displacement should proceed straight to ORIF.

Fracture of the hook (or hamulate) of the hamate
This rare injury occurs following a fall onto a dorsiflexed wrist, or when a player catches the ground or an object protruding from the ground, during the high-velocity phase of the swing, causing the racket or club handle to be forced against the hypothenar eminence.

Examination reveals pain, swelling and tenderness over the proximal hypothenar eminence. This fracture is frequently missed when investigated using plain X-rays, with oblique views being necessary to demonstrate the fracture. An axial CT scan is the best method if available.

Many texts will describe the treatment of choice as excision of the fragment; however, this procedure is actually very difficult and most will heal conservatively. Exogen (pulsed ultrasound) used 20 min/day for 6 weeks has been shown to be of benefit.

Scaphoid-lunate dissociation
This pathology is often associated with degenerative changes within the joint and presents in a similar group to those suffering problems of the triangular fibrocartilage complex (TFCC; see below), namely ice and field hockey players or gymnasts. Acute presentations may occur in any sport following a fall onto the dorsiflexed wrist.

The complaint is usually one of pain during activity, with some associated swelling. Examination demonstrates discomfort over the scapholunate joint, and the scaphoid shift test (radial deviation of the wrist with pressure over the scaphoid tuberosity) confirms the disruption.

'**Clenched fist views**' will demonstrate the separation of the two bones (Terry Thomas sign), while MRI will show a similar pattern but may demonstrate bone bruising.

Surgery is the treatment of choice, with a repair being undertaken in those injuries less than 6 months old.

Carpal dislocation
These injuries occur following forced hyperextension of the wrist. Injuries are associated with significant ligamentous disruption. The commonest presentations are lunate dislocation (dorsal or volar) or perilunar dislocation (lunate remains in fossa and carpus undergoes dorsal or volar dislocation). Median nerve compression is an accompanying complication of the former, whilst the latter is often associated with a scaphoid fracture. Surgical repair of these injuries with prolonged immobilization is the treatment of choice, with carpal instability and arthrosis being possible long-term sequelae.

Chronic wrist injuries

De Quervain's tenosynovitis

The abductor pollicis longus and extensor pollicis brevis tendons run in a synovial sheath passing beneath the lateral side of the extensor retinaculum. It is at this point that they can become inflamed, the usual cause being repetitive movements in, for example, racket sport players or activities such as rowing.

Examination often reveals both tenderness and crepitus at the level of the wrist, with Finkelstein's test – ulnar deviation of the wrist to produce pain – proving positive.

Investigations are not required as this is a clinical diagnosis.

Treatment includes the addressing of any biomechanical or technical factors alongside the usual physiotherapeutic modalities. Corticosteroid injection is useful in cases that are slow to resolve.

Intersection syndrome is a differential diagnosis of this condition, presenting as pain more proximally. The pathology is a bursitis at the point where the two above mentioned tendons cross the extensor carpi radialis tendons. It is common in sports such as rowing or kayaking (Fig. 5.4).

Nerve entrapment syndromes

Both the median and ulnar nerves are prone to entrapment in the wrist.

• **Median nerve entrapment at the wrist (carpal tunnel syndrome):** The median nerve runs in the forearm adherent to the flexor digitorum superficialis, and enters the wrist through the carpal tunnel, where compression can occur. Apart from sporting activities that can put pressure on this area (cycling is one of note), there are many systemic causes of carpal tunnel syndrome, including pregnancy, thyroid disease, and arthritic changes in the wrist itself. The complaint is often one of night pain, and paraesthesiae within the median nerve distribution, affecting the palmar aspect over the thumb and two-and-a-half fingers. Tinel's test is often positive (reproduces symptoms by percussing over carpal tunnel), as is Phalen's test (symptoms brought on by maximal palmar flexion of the wrist, held for 1 minute).

Nerve conduction studies will confirm the diagnosis, with treatment progressing from night splinting to corticosteroid injection and finally surgical decompression.

• **Ulnar nerve entrapment at the wrist:** A branch of the ulnar nerve passes between the hook of the hamate and the pisiform beneath the pisohamate ligament. Compression may occur here, especially in cyclists.

Examination reveals wasting and weakness within the interossei and adductor pollicis (positive Froment's sign). Altered sensation occurs over the little and ring fingers only, as the sensory supply to the skin over the hypothenar eminence and the dorsal aspect of the ulnar side of the hand is supplied by branches of the nerve that do not pass through the tunnel.

Changing the mechanics of the provoking activity, for example by a cyclist changing his or her grip, are first line in producing a cure.

Ulnar wrist pain

• **Disruption of the triangular fibrocartilage complex (TFCC)/articular disc:** This injury may be acute or chronic, and is usually associated with high-energy sports such as lacrosse and hockey, but also occurs in racket sports and golf.

Swelling and tenderness are noted around the medial side of the wrist joint; compressing the structure with ulnar deviation produces discomfort. This manoeuvre also differentiates it from other diagnoses. Magnetic resonance (MR) arthrography is the gold standard when investigating this condition. Acute tears may be repaired or debrided; chronic tears are not amenable to repair. Bracing may be of use in settling some of these cases.

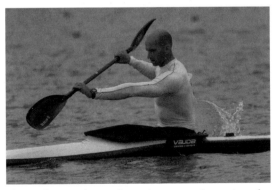

Fig. 5.4 Intersection syndrome is common in sports such as kayaking.

- **Tear to the extensor carpi ulnaris:** This is a not un-common differential diagnosis when presented with ulnar wrist pain. Diagnosis is made by distracting the ulnar-deviated wrist.
- **Ulnar abutment:** This may also present in a similar manner. It occurs when the ulna is longer than the radius. Ulnar deviation will reproduce symptoms. Shortening of the bone may be required.

Other chronic wrist injuries

Other wrist injuries that are of interest to the sports physician are those to the distal radio-ulnar joint and epiphyses. The former often occur as a result of ligamentous injuries in contact and racket sports; epiphyseal injuries are common in young gymnasts and are clearly demonstrated with plain X-ray films.

Ganglions are also a common presentation in the wrist at any age and may be treated with aspiration, although recurrence is common and surgical removal is often required if symptomatic.

Kienböck's disease may also present in the athlete as a swollen or painful wrist. The aetiology of this condition is uncertain and there may be no history of injury. The underlying pathology is one of avascular necrosis of the lunate. Early recognition is important if management is to be at all successful. It is a diagnosis that is frequently missed, although quite easily made, following plain X-rays.

Injuries of the hand

Fractures and dislocations

Metacarpal fractures

Metacarpal fractures occur usually as a result of a punch and so are common in contact sports. Fracture of the fifth metacarpal is frequently seen and is treated with cast immobilization or splinting, for 2–3 weeks.

Metacarpal fractures of the index, middle and ring fingers may present late, and as a lump felt by the athlete in the palm. If diagnosed at the time of injury, treatment is as above, although less angulation is accepted with the index and middle fingers due to the possibility of the above mentioned lump occurring as a consequence.

X-ray is sufficient to confirm the diagnosis and assess angulation and rotation.

Rotational alignment is the key and will dictate whether simple splinting or surgical fixation is necessary, with the index finger often requiring internal fixation for this reason.

An intra-articular fracture of the base of the first metacarpal (Bennett's fracture) should always be treated by surgical fixation and subsequent immobilization.

Phalangeal fractures

These fractures usually occur as a result of a ball impacting the finger or a rotational force. Sports with a high incidence of these injuries include basketball, netball, rugby and Australian rules football.

Treatment involves splinting the fracture. Again, as with fractures of the metacarpals, the degree of rotation is important and will decide whether internal fixation is required. Examining the fingers in flexion is a simple way of assessing this.

Interphalangeal dislocation

Dislocation occurs at both the proximal and distal interphalangeal joints (PIP and DIP), with a dorsal dislocation of the PIP joint being the most common presentation. Hyperextension occurring as a result of a ball hitting the end of the finger is the usual cause, and in most cases the dislocation is reduced on the field, although an X-ray should be performed afterwards to exclude a fracture. There is also risk of volar plate disruption following this injury, and therefore an open injury or any suggestion of the joint being locked or unstable, should be followed by referral to a hand surgeon for wash out and open repair of the structure.

Volar dislocations of both joints are less common; however, they frequently involve more serious injury to the joint and surrounding structures, so on-field reduction should not be attempted.

Ligament and tendon injuries

Medial (ulnar) collateral ligament of 1st metacarpophalangeal joint (skier's thumb)

Injury to this ligament is usually sustained by falling forwards onto an outstretched hand, whilst holding, for instance, a ski pole. It is also not uncommon in sports such as basketball, where the ball catches the thumb, which is forcibly abducted and hyperextended at the metacarpophalangeal (MCP) joint.

Examination reveals pain, swelling and localized tenderness, with discomfort reproduced when a valgus strain is applied to the joint. Excessive joint laxity may indicate a partial or complete tear of the ligament; the former requires immobilization through splinting or taping, whilst the latter should be referred for surgical repair not least because a 'Stener's lesion' (interposition of adductor aponeurosis within the joint) is a possible complication and would prevent ligamentous healing.

Mallet finger (extensor digitorum rupture)

The mechanism of this injury is one of a sudden axial load to the finger as may occur in sports such as basketball or cricket, causing forced flexion at the distal interphalangeal joint (DIP), resulting in a rupture of the extensor tendon attachment.

Examination reveals localized tenderness and loss of active DIP extension.

X-rays are required as the injury may be bony or tendinous, with significant bony involvement requiring ORIF. Off-the-shelf Mallet splints have been used for many years; however, these do not splint the joint in hyperextension and so lead to recurrence. The finger should be splinted in hyperextension using an aluminium splint for a minimum of six weeks and then reassessed.

Boutonnière deformity

This injury occurs when the central extensor slip is ruptured and the lateral bands subluxate. Again, it often occurs in ball-related sports, when the joint is forced into flexion.

Examination will reveal a deformity where the finger is classically flexed at the PIP joint and extended at the DIP joint.

Management consists of open repair, then protection of the repair in an extension splint, whilst mobilizing the DIP joint.

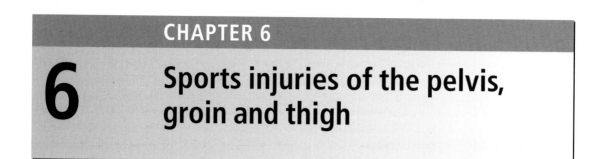

6 Sports injuries of the pelvis, groin and thigh

Anatomy of the hip, groin and thigh (Fig. 6.1)

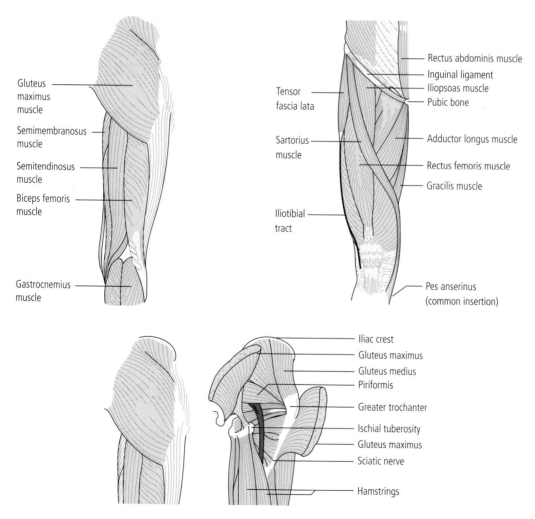

Gluteus maximus muscle

Semimembranosus muscle

Semitendinosus muscle

Biceps femoris muscle

Gastrocnemius muscle

Tensor fascia lata

Sartorius muscle

Iliotibial tract

Rectus abdominis muscle

Inguinal ligament

Iliopsoas muscle

Pubic bone

Adductor longus muscle

Rectus femoris muscle

Gracilis muscle

Pes anserinus (common insertion)

Iliac crest

Gluteus maximus

Gluteus medius

Piriformis

Greater trochanter

Ischial tuberosity

Gluteus maximus

Sciatic nerve

Hamstrings

Fig. 6.1 Muscles of the hip, groin and thigh region.

The groin's complex anatomical blend of nerves, vessels, musculotendinous origins and insertions, bursae and fascial layers is largely responsible for the diagnostic difficulties it poses for the sports physician.

The causes of groin pain are multiple and complex, presenting many diagnostic and treatment dilemmas, with sports such as soccer reporting injury rates as high as one in five of all competitors in any one year. There is, however, little scientific research to support many of the treatment protocols, further complicated by the fact that many diagnoses and treatments are both disputed and disagreed upon by the medical fraternity. A detailed anatomical knowledge is therefore required.

The epigastrium at T7, the umbilicus at T10 and the L1 dermatome described along a line proximal to the inguinal ligament, provide useful dermatomal landmarks.

Transversus abdominis (TA) forms the deep layer of the abdominal musculature, originating from structures including the lower six costal cartilages, the anterior two-thirds of the iliac crest and lateral third of the inguinal ligament and passing horizontally to a central insertion into the linea alba, stretching from the xiphoid process proximally to the symphysis pubis distally.

The lower portion produces a tendon, which 'conjoins' with fibres from the internal oblique forming the 'conjoint tendon', which inserts centrally into the linea alba and symphysis pubis.

The internal oblique forms the middle layer, overlying TA. It originates in part from the lumbar fascia and iliac crest, passing upwards at right angles to the external oblique and inserting over a wide area into the linea alba in exactly the same fashion as TA. It also inserts into the lower three ribs, with fibres passing backwards behind the spermatic cord to become the conjoint tendon as described.

Finally, external oblique forms the outer layer of the abdominal wall. The fibres originate from the last eight ribs, forming an aponeurosis that inserts in the same fashion as the previous layers into the linea alba, in addition to the anterior portion of the iliac crest, with its curved lower border becoming the inguinal ligament, opening medially as the superficial inguinal ring.

These muscles assist in flexion, rotation and lateral trunk flexion, also helping produce increased intra-abdominal pressure through the Valsalva manoeuvre.

Rectus abdominis lies most superficially and centrally, originating from the symphysis pubis and inserting into the xiphoid process and costal cartilages of ribs 5, 6 and 7. It is enclosed by the rectus sheath.

The hip joint localizes pain poorly, being supplied by articular branches from the obturator nerve, and pain often radiates into the anterior thigh and down to the knee.

Other important structures are tensor fascia lata, which originates from the iliac crest between the anterior superior iliac spine (ASIS) and the iliac tubercle and inserts into the iliotibial tract. The piriformis muscle is an external rotator of the thigh, originating from the bodies of S2, 3 and 4 anteriorly and inserting into the greater trochanter.

The thigh is divided into three compartments: anterior, medial and posterior.

Anterior compartment

This compartment contains several important structures. The sartorius muscle originates from the ASIS and inserts into the medial tibia as part of the common 'pes anserinus' tendon. Its actions are to flex, abduct and externally rotate the thigh at the hip, whilst flexing and internally rotating the leg at the knee. The iliopsoas originates from the transverse processes of T12 to L5, enters the thigh deep to the inguinal ligament, and inserts into the lesser trochanter. Its actions are to flex and internally rotate the thigh or alternatively to flex the trunk if the thigh is fixed.

Completing the important structures within this compartment are the rectus femoris originating from the AIIS, and the vastus medialis, intermedius and lateralis, which originate from the intertrochanteric line and medial lip of the linea aspera, anterolateral part of the femoral shaft and intertrochanteric line, and lateral lip of the linea aspera, respectively. These four structures combine to form the quadriceps tendon, inserting into the patella and collectively producing the powerful quadriceps femoris muscle group, which extends the knee. The rectus femoris also acts as a hip flexor.

Medial compartment

Structures of importance are gracilis, originating from the inferior pubic and ischial rami, and forming part of the pes anserinus common insertion into the tibia and acting by adducting the thigh at the hip and flexing the leg at the knee. The adductor muscle group, consisting of longus, brevis and magnus, take their origins in that order, from the pubis anteromedially, through to the ischial tuberosity posteriorly. Their main action is to adduct the thigh at the hip joint, whilst also assisting in external rotation. Additionally the hamstring portion of magnus extends the thigh at the hip and could be included within the posterior compartment.

Posterior compartment

This compartment contains the hamstring group. The biceps femoris has two origins, its long head attaching to the ischial tuberosity, whilst the short head arises from the linea aspera and lateral supracondylar ridge of the femur. It inserts into the head of the fibula, flexing and externally rotating the leg at the knee, whilst also extending the thigh at the hip. Semitendinosus also originates from the ischial tuberosity via a common tendon with biceps femoris, inserting into the medial tibia, as the last of the three elements that comprise the pes anserinus. Semimembranosus completes the group, originating from the ischial tuberosity and inserting into the posteromedial surface of the tibial condyle, also forming the oblique popliteal ligament. These two muscles both act by producing flexion and internal rotation of the leg at the knee, whilst also extending the thigh at the hip.

The sciatic nerve is the largest nerve in the body and a frequent cause of symptomatology, so an understanding of its anatomy is important. Originating from the sacral plexus (L4,5, S1–3), it exits the pelvis through the greater sciatic notch. In a minority the nerve then passes through the piriformis, where problems can arise. It exits the buttock by passing deep to the long head of biceps, another area of concern, and descends in the thigh beneath biceps femoris and semimembranosus before dividing into the tibial and common peroneal nerves.

Acute presentation of thigh and groin pain

Musculotendinous injuries

Many of the structures described above within the groin and upper leg are commonly involved in acute thigh and groin pain, and the important presentations are detailed below.

Adductor-related pain

Presentation
This is a common finding in most twisting and turning sports. The athlete complains of a sudden onset of pain within the groin region.

Diagnosis
Palpation elicits pain at the adductor teno-osseous junction or locally within the adductor muscle belly. Passive abduction and resisted adduction, undertaken with the knee and hip initially flexed and then straightened, throughout various ranges to stress all elements of the adductor group, also causes discomfort.

Further investigations are not usually necessary, but if available, diagnostic ultrasound can be used to demonstrate muscular disruption in those presenting with muscular or musculotendinous junction symptomatology. Discomfort at the teno-osseous junction is more difficult to delineate with ultrasound and is better demonstrated on MRI; however, this is unnecessary unless the condition is failing to resolve.

Management
The use of nonsteroidal anti-inflammatory drugs (NSAIDs) is indicated acutely, with the usual rehabilitation protocol being followed (see Chapter 18). Eccentric strengthening predominates in these cases as the athlete progresses. Corticosteroid injection may be of help in nonresponsive cases, which usually involve the teno-osseous junction.

An alternative pathology should be considered here if the presentation is more insidious or recurrent, especially in cases involving older players, where symptoms are more likely to originate from an adductor tendinosis. As with other tendons, such as Achilles, tendonotic pathology is becoming in-

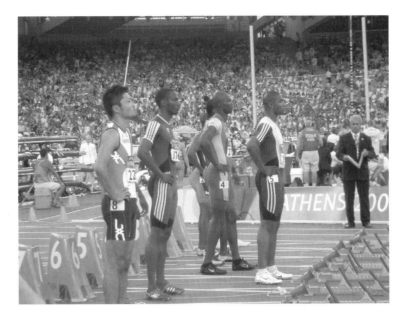

Fig. 6.2 Acute hamstring injuries are common in sprinters.

creasingly recognized as a reason for nonresolution of symptoms. Research has pointed towards eccentric strengthening regimes as being the cornerstone of managing these conditions, with recovery times being prolonged, often taking up to 4 months.

In cases that still fail to resolve, adductor tenotomy may be considered as a final measure.

Quadriceps-related pain

Presentation

The quadriceps group (see 'Anatomy' above), like the hamstrings, is frequently injured as a result of the combination of eccentric loading with these muscles spanning two joints. Injuries, not surprisingly, are common in sports that involve kicking. Adult populations may rarely present with an avulsion injury of the ASIS at the attachment of sartorius.

Rectus femoris injuries tend to present as mid-belly muscle tears, whilst younger age groups are more likely to present with an apophysitis or avulsion of the rectus femoris from the anterior inferior iliac spine.

Diagnosis

Clinical examination usually confirms the diagnosis. However, X-rays or ultrasound will give confirmation if an avulsion injury is suspected. Ultrasound

will also help to confirm the level of disruption following muscular injury and is useful in assessing any haematoma formation or the possible development of myositis ossificans, an occasional sequela following a contusion and subsequent development of an intramuscular haematoma in the quadriceps region.

Management

The usual rehab protocols are followed, taking care to ensure that the player is symptom free before he or she resumes kicking, as recurrence is not uncommon in cases that are inadequately rehabilitated.

Hamstring pain

Presentation

Pain in the posterior thigh region can prove more of a diagnostic dilemma than anterior thigh pain, because of the large number of structures that refer pain to this area (see Chapter 9).

Acute hamstring injuries, however, tend to present with a classical history in which the athlete is forced to pull up suddenly, usually whilst sprinting or running at pace (Fig. 6.2). Depending on the severity of the injury, various levels of debility occur due to the ensuing muscle spasm (see 'Track and field' in Chapter 16)

Diagnosis

Clinical examination will reveal the extent of the injury, with more severe injuries, often described as grade 3, demonstrating a palpable defect in some cases. Hamstring stretches will provoke pain, as will resisted testing, with the athlete often able to localize pain to the injured area.

Ultrasound is useful in assessing injury severity, and, in deeper tears, the presence of an associated haematoma.

Injuries occurring at the hamstring origin can prove more intractable and recovery is more prolonged. Avulsion injuries are not uncommon in this area; however, they are a more frequent finding in adolescents (see Chapter 12). X-rays will highlight them, although they are often easily visualized using ultrasound.

Management

The usual guidelines are followed. However, accelerated programmes have recently proved quite successful in reducing time lost to sport and are described in Chapter 18. The only downside to this approach is the possible increase in recurrence following this type of regime.

Avulsion injuries follow a more protracted recovery. Intervention is not usually necessary unless the avulsed fragment is widely separated and the athlete is failing to progress (usually an adolescent); surgical reattachment may then occasionally be necessary.

One possible complication of hamstring injuries that fail to resolve is the progression to a chronic, scarred state. Referring back to the anatomy, it was noted that the sciatic nerve runs close to the long head of biceps, and it is here that problems can arise, with the nerve becoming entangled in the scar tissue. In some cases surgical intervention is even required.

Other muscular injuries

Presentation

The iliopsoas is a powerful hip flexor. Iliopsoas bursitis and tendonitis is a common diagnosis used to describe the presentation of deep groin pain and indeed is correct in some, but most definitely not all cases labelled as such, with true psoas bursitis in fact being relatively rare.

The athlete often complains of a deep, nonspecific groin pain, which may have arisen acutely, but often presents with a gradual onset.

Diagnosis

Care must be taken not to overcall this as misdiagnosis can lead to the neglect of more serious hip pathology such as pelvic or hip stress fractures.

Deep palpation may prove helpful. However, resisted testing is often more specific and can be undertaken in a number of ways. Resisted hip flexion with the hip in extension will reproduce symptoms, as may testing with the athlete supine and the legs held in extension and slight external rotation to remove the action of rectus femoris. Lunging may also reproduce symptoms (Fig. 6.3).

Ultrasound is the investigation of choice for those resistant to initial treatment modalities.

Management

The usual approach of stretching and strengthening generally produces a resolution of symptoms, with NSAIDs also proving useful.

Persisting tightness within the psoas tendon may be the reason some fail to settle, with excessive shortening sometimes leading to the condition known as 'snapping hip'; ongoing pain in this instance is due to the tight tendon flipping across the front of the joint during active hip flexion. The iliotibial band and hip capsule are two other structures that should be considered in this diagnosis.

Other acute causes of hip pain

Labral tear

A tear of the acetabular labrum can present as an acute cause of hip pain (but equally commonly is a result of gradual deterioration of the structure over a long career). Not uncommon in twisting, turning and kicking sports such as soccer, the history is usually one of a tearing sensation as the player twists or extends the leg, resulting in immediate discomfort. The injury is often not severe enough to remove the player from the game; however, symptoms then progress over the next few weeks. Examination often reveals localized discomfort on direct palpation over

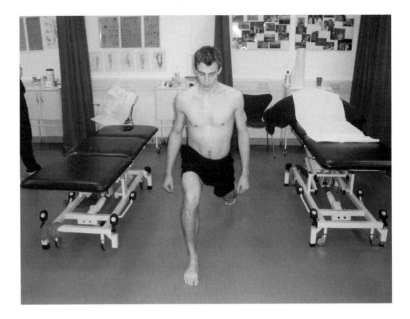

Fig. 6.3 The lunge.

the joint, with pain being reproduced by undertaking a quadrant test (Fig. 6.4), which compresses the structure in much the same way as the adduction stress test ('empty can' test) does with glenoid labral tears.

Some may resolve with restriction of all aggravating activities. However, in the professional sportsperson, hip arthroscopy and debridement is often necessary to produce a cure.

Chondral injury

Damage to the articular cartilage of the femoral head does occur, but it is a significantly less frequent occurrence than noted in, for instance, the knee and ankle joints. The injury can be acute or acute on chronic, with arthroscopic chondroplasty being the treatment of choice. Unfortunately, early osteoarthritic change will follow.

Slipped capital femoral epiphysis (SCFE)

The diagnosis of slipped capital femoral epiphysis would be the likely pathology in the adolescent child, more commonly found in the female population. There is also an increased association with obesity or following a significant growth spurt, with 25% presenting bilaterally (see Chapter 12).

Chronic presentation of thigh and groin pain

Whilst many conditions present acutely in this region, there are as many if not more conditions with a more insidious onset. Chronic groin and leg pain test the clinician's clinical acumen to its limits.

The most common conditions, sportsman's hernia and osteitis pubis, will be described first, with the common adductor tendonopathies having already been discussed alongside their acute presentations.

Sportsman's hernia

Presentation

This is often referred to as Gilmore's groin in the UK, or as South Australia groin 'down under'. Both the diagnosis and treatment of this condition are contentious issues. Most cases arise in sports such as soccer and rugby, where high-velocity twisting and turning appears to be the aggravating factor. Onset of symptoms is usually insidious, but can be acute, with the athlete initially complaining of a dull ache within the lower abdomen or groin, associated with exercise, particularly if involving twisting, sprinting and kicking. Symptoms progress over a variable timeframe, with exercises such as sit-ups causing discomfort, until even coughing, sneezing or turning in bed becomes uncomfortable. Eventually rest pain, stiffness and adductor weakness become persistent findings. Rest often improves symptoms temporarily; however, they classically and frustratingly return almost immediately on resuming the aggravating exercise, even after prolonged periods.

Diagnosis

Examination may reveal pain on scrotal invagination, and resisted tests such as the 'Direct Stress Examination' – consisting of palpation of the lower abdomen with the feet raised 15 cm – may prove uncomfortable. There is often tenderness on palpation over the distal portion of the inguinal ligament, and the quadrant or 'fade' test may produce discomfort, presumably due to compression of the damaged tissues (Fig. 6.4). In summary, no one test in isolation is diagnostic, with the overall clinical picture being important.

Disagreement also exists regarding the correct investigative protocols. Some advocate herniogram, a procedure producing positive results in almost as many asymptomatic groins as symptomatic ones. MRI is becoming more popular, with specialist centres offering specific groin protocols. It is, however, the combination of these radiological and clinical investigations in experienced hands that will produce the most accurate outcomes.

Management

Many will progress to surgery, with rehabilitation often proving unsuccessful and certainly in the case of professional football, too protracted. This begs the question as to whether it is the enforced rest that produces the cure.

The pathology varies, with some describing a defect in the conjoint tendon or a disruption of its insertion into the pubic tubercle. Findings may be of a bulging in the transversalis fascia, with weakened, dilated external inguinal rings, often described as 'posterior wall weakness'. One suspects that at surgery the pathology is not always immediately evident; however, the results tend to support the intervention, with most returning rapidly to sport and recurrences proving infrequent, although there still appears to be little consensus between surgeons.

Procedures also vary, with some surgeons using a mesh to reinforce the posterior wall, whilst others describe a detailed anatomical repair of the above mentioned structures.

In many, abnormal findings are noted incidentally on the asymptomatic side and as it is not infrequent for a similar problem to occur on the other side soon

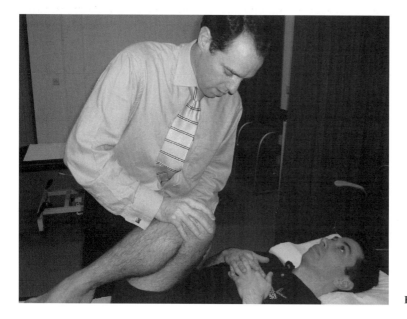

Fig. 6.4 The quadrant test.

after surgery, a number of surgeons will operate on the asymptomatic side at the same time.

Various rehabilitation regimes have been described, but in general the aim is the rapid return of the athlete to sport. Gentle exercise such as walking commences within 24–48 hours of surgery, running being introduced by the end of the first week, sprinting by week 3 and a return to competition within 4–5 weeks, depending on the extent of surgical repair necessary.

Osteitis pubis

Presentation

First described as far back as 1932, this term is often used as a diagnostic label for vague, insidious groin pain, in a similar manner to that in which 'chondromalacia patella' was used to encompass all causes of anterior knee pain and in some circles still is! The history is one of a gradual onset of clinical symptoms consisting of suprapubic pain, often with a radiation into the lower abdomen and inner thigh region and occasionally even into the scrotum, with sports involving running or kicking predominating.

Diagnosis

Examination reveals tenderness over the symphysis pubis, with hip movements being limited, particularly in abduction, in almost all cases.

X-rays demonstrate the classical radiological findings of erosions and sclerosis of the symphysis pubis, described as the 'moth eaten appearance'. Stalk views will sometimes highlight instability, with greater than 2 mm of movement in the joint being deemed significant.

Other pathologies may be confused with this condition and so careful examination is paramount.

Management

Standard treatment is of removal from the aggravating activity, which seems initially necessary in all cases. NSAIDs and hip stretches are then often advocated; however, a symptom-free return to sport in some cases can take up to 6 months.

Corticosteroid injection into the symphyseal cleft proves beneficial with some, and certain studies suggest that early referral and treatment in this way may indeed significantly reduce recovery time in this protracted but self-limiting condition.

Stress fractures

Presentation

Stress fractures of the femoral neck and pubic rami are a worrying and common finding, particularly in female distance runners. The oestrogen-sensitive long trabecular and flat bones are those affected by low oestrogenic conditions experienced by some amenorrhoeic athletes, hence their susceptibility to developing stress fractures. They include the superior and inferior margins of the femoral neck, the symptoms being of groin pain often radiating into the anterior thigh or knee; stress fractures of the superior margin of the femoral neck are treated as an emergency because of their high possibility of progression to fracture.

Other sites commonly affected are the pubic rami, usually inferior, and the femoral shaft. These diagnoses should always be considered when faced with a history of unresolved groin pain, further supported by suspicious characteristics such as pain on loading with activities such as hopping, or the red flag of night pain.

Diagnosis

The history will point to the diagnosis, and examination may reproduce pain in more advanced cases on flexion and internal rotation of the hip. Less advanced cases may require activities such as single leg hopping to reproduce symptoms.

If any discomfort is elicited on clinical examination and the condition is suspected to be anything more than an early stress reaction, X-rays should be taken. If negative, MRI scan will then confirm suspicions. An isotope bone scan is also diagnostic but is used less frequently now.

Management

A more aggressive approach is taken than with other stress fractures. In the case of compression fractures (i.e. inferior margin of femoral neck), in the presence of a normal X-ray, non-weight-bearing rest is advised until the athlete is asymptomatic. This may take up to 6 weeks before weight bearing and exercise are gradually reintroduced over the next few months. If a fracture line is visible, then bed rest is enforced until fracture healing is demonstrated radiographically and the athlete is symptom free.

Distraction fractures of the superior margin require even more aggressive attention because of their tendency to progress to complete fracture, which often displaces resulting in nonunion and avascular necrosis.

Stress fractures of the pubic rami are treated in much the same way as any other, with relative rest and restriction of the aggravating activity until symptoms resolve.

Nerve entrapment syndromes

Presentation
There are four nerve entrapment syndromes that cause symptoms in this region.

The **ilioinguinal nerve** originates from the lumbar plexus, deriving its supply from L1 and entering the thigh via the superficial inguinal ring. Entrapment produces an area of pain or paraesthesiae, noted around the genitalia and inside of the thigh.

The **genitofemoral nerve** may also be affected, again emerging as a branch of the lumbar plexus with a root derivation of L1/2. It can be associated with symptoms experienced inferior to the inguinal ligament in the midline.

The **obturator nerve** may also become entrapped. It originates from the lumbar plexus with a root derivation of L2–4, and runs through the obturator foramen, at which point it splits, with the anterior branch supplying the skin of the medial thigh, whilst also giving motor branches to the gracilis and adductor longus and brevis, in addition to supplying the hip joint.

Entrapment of the **lateral cutaneous nerve of the thigh** is a common presentation in nonsporting populations. However, sports such as rowing or cycling can produce compression. It supplies the skin over the lateral thigh.

Piriformis syndrome

It was noted in the anatomical description that in some individuals the sciatic nerve passes through the piriformis muscle. Occasionally this can result in neurological irritation of the nerve with buttock and posterior leg pain.

The piriformis also appears to be a very irritable muscle, and the normal discomfort noted by most when palpated is exacerbated in some individuals, the muscle becoming restricted and shortened, with symptoms being reproduced on direct palpation or resisted testing. Quadrant stretches and soft tissue work will produce a resolution of symptoms.

This is probably a syndrome that is again much overdiagnosed.

Other causes of groin and thigh pain

The iliotibial band has been mentioned as a cause of symptoms around the knee, but it can also produce similar problems around the greater trochanter in association with the trochanteric bursa. Treatment consists of stretches and myofascial release techniques, whilst a nonresolving trochanteric bursitis may require injection of corticosteroid.

Both irritable hip and Perthes disease would be a consideration in those presenting between 2 and 10 years, the latter more frequently seen in boys, with 15% being bilateral.

Osteoarthritis is an expected presentation in older age groups, but is also increasing in frequency in the younger professional sportsperson, whilst the possibility of infection and avascular necrosis should never be forgotten due to their disastrous consequences.

Intra-abdominal pathology, including that of the appendix, prostate and many gynaecological conditions, should always be considered, also remembering that testicular tumours are particularly common in this younger population.

The sporting pelvis and groin will remain one of the sports practitioner's greatest challenges because of the multiple above mentioned pathologies, and it is only by considering these many possible diagnoses that successful management will be achieved.

7 Sports injuries of the knee and lower leg

The knee joint

Knee injuries are responsible for up to half of all time lost to sporting activity. Although occurring less frequently than thigh injuries in soccer or lateral ankle ligament sprains in general – the latter being the most commonly sustained sporting injury – prolonged rehabilitation is often required, with 25% still having problems up to a year later. Early and accurate diagnosis is therefore essential, enabling appropriate rehabilitation or speedy referral. Clinical examination in expert hands has been shown to be as reliable as high-tech radiological investigation, the decision on whether to progress to arthroscopic examination often being made without resorting to costly imaging such as MRI.

Injuries once thought of as 'career ending' can now be treated successfully, although outcomes are still largely dependent on help being sought from specialist centres.

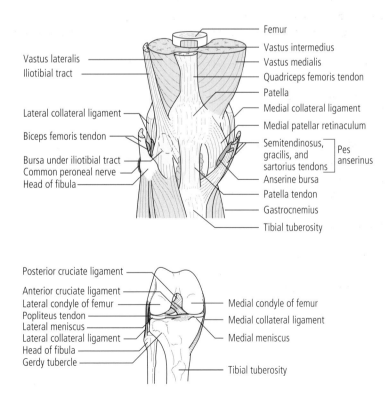

Fig. 7.1 Anatomy of the knee.

Anatomy (Fig. 7.1)

The knee joint is a synovial hinge joint involving the articulation between the femur and tibia, the patella also forming a separate articulation with the femur. The capsule surrounds the medial, lateral and posterior part of the joint, with its absence anteriorly allowing the presence of the synovial membrane to be visualized as the suprapatellar bursa.

Important structures include the menisci, which are two crescents of fibrocartilage attached to the capsule by their lateral margins. The medial meniscus is more fixed and as a consequence is the more commonly injured of the two.

The medial collateral ligament attaches proximally to the medial femoral condyle and distally to the tibia, at least two fingerbreadths below the medial joint line.

The anterior cruciate ligament is intracapsular, although extrasynovial. It attaches anteriorly to the intercondylar area of the tibia and posteriorly to the lateral femoral condyle, on its posteromedial side; that is, it passes anteromedial to posterolateral. Conversely, the posterior cruciate ligament passes in an opposite manner from an insertion on the tibial plateau in an anterior direction, again inserting into the femoral condyle.

Laterally the popliteus tendon originates from the lateral side of the lateral femoral condyle within the joint capsule, running alongside the lateral meniscus, but not usually attaching to it. The insertion of the muscle is into the posterior surface of the tibia, passing downwards and medially.

The lateral collateral ligament attaches proximally to the lateral femoral epicondyle, inserting distally into the fibula head. The iliotibial band originates from the iliac tubercle and inserts into the lateral tibial condyle, consisting of a lateral thickening of the fascia lata.

Acute knee injuries

Common acute knee injuries include:
- medial or lateral meniscal tears;
- anterior cruciate ligament (ACL) rupture;
- medial collateral ligament (MCL) injury;
- posterior cruciate ligament (PCL) rupture;
- patellar dislocation;
- articular cartilage damage.

A detailed history provides the most important diagnostic information when dealing with an acute knee injury, particularly as examination may be difficult in a grossly swollen, painful knee. The mechanism of injury may provide the physician with a good indicator as to the possible structures damaged. Any accompanying 'pop' is suggestive of an ACL injury. The degree and time of onset of swelling is an important diagnostic clue. When a haemarthrosis is present, the swelling is usually considerable and occurs within the first 1–2 hours after injury. The likely causes of a haemarthrosis are ACL rupture or patellar dislocation. An effusion that develops over the 24 hours after injury is a feature of meniscal injuries. There is usually little or no swelling associated with medial ligament injuries.

Meniscal injuries

Presentation

Meniscal injuries are more commonly seen in sports such as soccer, rugby and netball as a result of the forces exerted on the joint as the player twists and turns. The fixed medial meniscus is most frequently injured, being torn when the player rotates on a flexed knee with the foot firmly planted. Immediate pain and debility follow, with swelling occurring gradually over a period of about 12–24 hours, in contrast to the immediate swelling associated with a haemarthrosis as described above. An occasional exception to this rule is a tear to the vascular outer third of the meniscus, which may bleed into the joint.

Giving way and pain during weight-bearing flexion are common complaints, with locking (i.e. 5–10° of fixed flexion) occurring in a minority (although indicating urgent surgical intervention).

Diagnosis

Examination will often reveal a small to moderate-sized effusion, with joint line tenderness being present in the region of the tear; as 70–80% of meniscal tears are of the posterior horn of the medial meniscus, the tenderness is usually noted around the posteromedial joint line.

Passive knee flexion usually reproduces the pain, symptoms being further exacerbated when the lower leg is externally rotated in this position. Hyperextension often produces discomfort, and in experienced hands these findings are usually sufficient to make the diagnosis.

McMurray's (flexion/rotation) test is still frequently used although its usefulness is questionable. Pain can be reproduced on squatting if passive flexion is inconclusive. The presence of a meniscal cyst over the lateral joint line indicates a degenerative tear of the lateral meniscus in as many as 90% of cases.

The diagnosis of meniscal injury is a clinical one and investigations are rarely required. The schools of thought relating to the appropriate investigation of suspected meniscal injury vary and it is a much debated subject at this time. The use of arthrography declined with the advent of MRI, which was proclaimed as a breakthrough in noninvasive diagnosis. However, as previously mentioned, a meniscal injury is a clinical diagnosis confirmed on examination, which when undertaken by a specialist in the field, has been shown to produce a high diagnostic accuracy. In inexperienced hands, attempts to achieve a diagnosis in borderline cases by using imaging can result in large numbers of false-positive MRI scans, leading to an increase in arthroscopic examination rather than a reduction.

Management

At arthroscopy a decision will be made regarding the appropriateness of meniscal suturing or partial meniscectomy (Chapter 16, Soccer).

Rehabilitation involving improving range of motion and strengthening exercises is commenced as soon as pain allows in the postoperative period. Weight bearing progresses from non-weight bearing (NWB) to full weight bearing (FWB) over a variable 0–6-week period depending on the intervention necessary. Suturing of a tear is a definite indicator for NWB for 6 weeks (therefore check with the operating surgeon).

An increased incidence of premature osteoarthritic changes has been noted in those suffering medial meniscal injuries in their early twenties. Chondral damage occurring either at the time of injury or as a consequence of the meniscal damage may be responsible. Preservation of as much of the damaged cartilage as possible, particularly following lateral meniscal tears, is important, with long-term outcome being poor following meniscectomy. Progression is often quite rapid, with degenerative changes developing within the lateral compartment and not uncommonly causing a premature end to a sporting career.

Chondral damage, as previously mentioned, often accompanies meniscal injuries or occurs subsequent to them, with chondroplasty and microfracture being two commonly used interventions aimed at improving outcome. Recent techniques such as chondral grafting and chondrocyte culture are becoming increasingly popular; however, more research is required before their success becomes evident.

Ligamentous injuries

Anterior cruciate ligament

Presentation

The action of the anterior cruciate ligament (ACL) is to prevent anterior displacement of the tibia on the femur. Injury usually occurs when a valgus force is applied to a flexed knee with the foot planted in external rotation (Fig. 7.2). Hyperextension of the internally rotated leg is a less common mechanism.

This mechanism of injury alongside the athlete's account of an associated 'pop' or 'snap', followed by immediate pain and a rapid onset of swelling (haemarthrosis) within 1–2 hours, is diagnostic. Occasional contradictions occur as acute 'on-field' treatment improves, with more ACL ruptures presenting with only moderate swelling, probably due to the early intervention of RICE (rest, ice, compression, elevation). Seventy percent of haemarthroses are caused by ACL rupture, with the majority of the other 30% being the result of osteochondral fractures

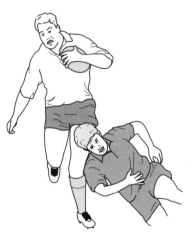

Fig. 7.2 Mechanism of injury in anterior cruciate ligament (ACL) rupture. Valgus force to the flexed knee with the foot fixed.

or tears of the vascular outer third of the medial meniscus.

Diagnosis

Acute examination can be difficult if swelling has already occurred. A positive Lachman's test helps confirm the diagnosis and is the most appropriate examination (Fig. 7.3). The pivot-shift test is sometimes used, but has a tendency to produce discomfort.

The ACL is often injured in association with other structures such as the medial meniscus, medial collateral ligament and posterior oblique ligament, injury to all four being described in the age-old Irish tradition as O'Donaghue's triad (Fig. 7.4)! A Segond fracture (a fracture of the tibial plateau) is also an occasional finding.

MRI is often used, especially in professional sport, for confirmation. However, this should really be a diagnosis made very much on the history and examination findings.

Management

Conservative management was not uncommon 15 years ago and is an option in the recreational athlete. However, surgical repair appears to be indicated in all those whose intent is to return to high-level sport.

Two methods are used to reconstruct the ACL using either the middle portion of the patellar tendon or the semitendinosus tendon as graft material. Repair can be undertaken either immediately or at 3–6 weeks, this decision being influenced by the symptomatology on presentation. If the athlete

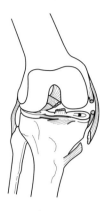

Fig. 7.4 O'Donoghue's triad. Rupture of medial collateral and anterior cruciate ligaments with tear of medial meniscus, and injury to posterior oblique ligament.

demonstrates full extension and a minimal effusion (i.e 'a quiet knee') then repair can be undertaken immediately. A block to extension and large effusion would suggest delaying until function improves, as outcome is adversely affected when surgery is undertaken in the symptomatic knee.

Following reconstruction, rehabilitation progresses over a 6-month period, culminating in a return to sport. Accelerated programmes have been used, often at a high cost, with cautionary tales recounted of graft rupture on the first day of competition. A sensible approach should therefore be adopted, allowing the graft adequate time to revascularize and strengthen. This will also ensure that the individual has regained adequate proprioception, undertaken late at 3–6 months, and sufficient strength, to produce the dynamic stability required.

Posterior cruciate ligament

Presentation

Posterior cruciate ligament rupture usually occurs following a direct impact to the tibia, just below the flexed knee. It is common in equestrian pursuits and rugby. There may be a feeling of instability but often no effusion, as a result of it being extrasynovial.

Diagnosis

Examination of the knee may reveal a posterior sag, with loss of the palpable prominence of the tibial plateau medially helping in less obvious cases (see Fig. 7.1). X-rays may help by demonstrating an avulsion

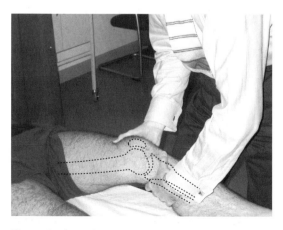

Fig. 7.3 Lachman's test.

of the PCL's tibial attachment, more commonly noted in adolescents.

Symptoms are often minimal, resulting in the diagnosis being missed – it has been shown that as many as 30% of professional rugby players have an undiagnosed rupture.

Management
Management tends to be conservative as the dysfunction associated with this injury is significantly less than that experienced following an ACL rupture.

Rehabilitation focuses initially on quadriceps strengthening, isolated hamstring exercises being an absolute contraindication during the first 6 weeks. Closed kinetic chain exercises are then incorporated, so allowing hamstring strengthening whilst protecting the ligament from excessive posterior tibial translation.

Surgical repair is, however, now being increasingly undertaken, although cases should be very carefully selected before intervention is decided upon, as a significant change in outcome has yet to be demonstrated.

Medial collateral ligament
Presentation
The medial collateral ligament (MCL), whose anatomy is described earlier, is more commonly injured than the LCL, with the classical history being that of a valgus force to the knee or a twisting injury, that is, external rotation combined with a valgus force – a common mechanism of injury encountered in skiing. As with the ACL, associated injuries are not uncommon.

Diagnosis
Inspection of the knee will demonstrate no effusion. The medial side of the joint is stressed in full extension and then in 10–30° of flexion, a position in which the knee is less stable, to demonstrate laxity or reproduce symptoms. Grade 1 and 2 tears commonly occur at the femoral attachment (i.e. 3 cm from the joint line), producing tenderness on palpation and localized discomfort on stressing the joint, in contrast to the often painless examination noted following complete disruption because of the severing of neural structures. Tears are often graded as shown in Box 7.1.

MRI is the investigation of choice in more severe cases, both to help grade the injury and exclude as-

---

> **Box 7.1** Grading of tears
>
> Grade 1   Minor tear/sprain (no laxity)
> Grade 2   Partial tear/sprain (stable in extension, lax at 30°)
> Grade 3   Total disruption

---

sociated damage to other structures, such as the ACL or medial meniscus.

Management
Management is conservative if dealing with an isolated injury. Grade 1 injuries are rehabilitated with a graduated programme of strengthening and increased range of movement (ROM) over 3–4 weeks. Grade 2/3 injuries are treated more conservatively, with a limited motion knee brace being used over the first 4 weeks, restricting the last 20–30° of extension. Recovery is obviously more prolonged and can take up to 10 weeks, depending on severity of injury.

Patellar dislocation or subluxation
Presentation
Patellar dislocation or subluxation typically occurs following a blow to the patella, for instance during a rugby tackle. It often relocates spontaneously, making the history all important and the diagnosis more difficult. The patella dislocates laterally, with the player recounting a feeling of the knee 'going out' and giving way, followed by acute pain and disability.

Diagnosis
Examination reveals tenderness and an effusion, with the patella even remaining dislocated in a few cases.

The 'patella apprehension test', in which pressure is applied to the medial side of the patella forcing it laterally, will also exacerbate symptoms and is diagnostic in recurrent cases. Recurrence can follow an initial injury but is preventable if the knee is adequately rehabilitated. X-rays should be taken to exclude an associated osteochondral fracture.

Management
Rehabilitation concentrates on patellofemoral stabilization in much the same way as is undertaken in cases of anterior knee pain, with taping being used in

the initial stages to protect the joint. Persistent symptoms would be an indication for arthroscopic examination, to exclude any associated chondral damage.

This condition may also occur spontaneously, usually presenting in young girls and often requiring surgical intervention if stabilization fails to occur following an intensive strengthening regime.

Lateral collateral ligament sprain

Injury to the lateral collateral ligament, which is most easily palpated in the 'figure of four' position (Fig. 7.5), is less common than that of the MCL, occurring following a varus force to the medial side of the knee.

Coronary (meniscotibial) ligament sprain

Coronary (meniscotibial) ligament sprains present in the older sportsperson, triggered by excessive rotation. Joint line tenderness can sometimes be confused with meniscal lesions. However, corticosteroid injection often produces rapid resolution of symptoms.

Overuse injuries of the knee

Anterior knee pain

Anterior knee pain is a common presentation within sports injury clinics, with numerous causes. Chondromalacia patellae, which is often given erroneously as a diagnosis, is in reality an uncommon pathological finding.

Patellofemoral joint pain

Presentation

Patellofemoral joint pain, sometimes called patellofemoral pain syndrome (PFPS) or medial or lateral patella pressure syndrome, is by far the commonest cause of anterior knee pain, with an increased incidence in runners and females. The presentation is one of retropatellar pain often accompanied by giving way, with symptoms worsened by downhill loading. The 'cinema sign', so called because pain occurs following prolonged sitting with the knee bent, is often reported.

A combination of tight lateral retinacular structures alongside weak medial structures results in maltracking and dysfunction within the patellofemoral joint and is responsible for the condition. Poor flexibility within certain muscle groups, especially hamstrings, gastrocnemius and soleus, often contributes to the overall picture and should be attended to.

A number of contributing biomechanical factors are noted below:

1 Malalignment syndrome is often present in women, with an increased Q angle, i.e. greater than the normal range of 15–20°, exerting forces on the patella, thereby increasing lateral translation and so aggravating the joint.
2 Excessive pronation (Fig. 7.6).
3 Leg length discrepancy of any significance should be corrected. Inappropriate training regimes may be implicated and even the inadvertent wearing of heel raises may aggravate symptoms.

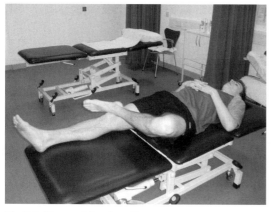

Fig. 7.5 'Figure of four' position.

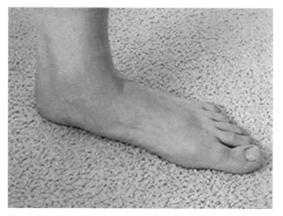

Fig. 7.6 Pronated foot with pes planus.

Diagnosis

Examination is often unremarkable, with no obvious effusion and a full range of pain-free motion, both actively and passively. Positive signs are usually found on palpation, when tenderness is often elicited under the medial or lateral patellar facets. Pain is more likely to be reproduced on encouraging the patient to actively load the knee in 20–30° of flexion. Inspection often reveals poor muscle definition in the vastus medialis obliquus (VMO), with poor control easily demonstrated by instructing the athlete to undertake a half squat.

Management

Management centres around three principles. The correction of any of the above biomechanical factors such as malalignment, strengthening of the medial structures such as VMO, using rehabilitative regimes including exercises such as single leg squats, with the use of biofeedback equipment if available and stretching of the lateral structures.

Taping may help during the rehabilitation period (Fig. 7.7) with its purpose being to produce symptomatic relief to allow rehabilitation to progress. Its action is thought to be more through increased proprioceptive feedback than providing mechanical support.

Useful adjuncts to achieving the above may be self-mobilization of tight lateral retinacular and iliotibial band structures. Excessive pronation should be corrected with the use of orthotics (Fig. 7.8) whilst neoprim supports containing a patellar stabilizer may be beneficial. NSAIDs are often helpful in the acute phase.

Surgical intervention is a last resort, with the vast majority settling following appropriate rehabilitation. If symptoms are intractable then a lateral release can be undertaken. This is now performed arthroscopically, with intensive physiotherapy being an absolute requirement, to prevent excessive scarring postoperatively. Studies vary, but show 75% to be symptom free at 7 years.

Patellar tendinopathy

Presentation

Patellar tendon problems are commonly associated with jumping activities, and so have a relatively high

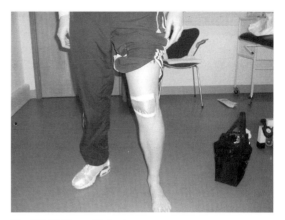

Fig. 7.7 McConnell's taping.

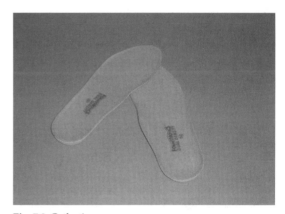

Fig. 7.8 Orthotics.

incidence in athletic field events and basketball, also occurring less frequently in sports such as soccer and ice hockey. Aetiological hypotheses suggest a condition that may be due to an abnormal healing response (Chapter 8, Achilles tendinosis). Whether there is a genetic predisposition is as yet unclear; however, advanced changes have been demonstrated in athletes as young as 17 or 18, a finding that also questions the labelling of tendinosis as a degenerative process. This is a separate entity from the acute presentation of patellar tendonitis, commonly known as 'jumper's knee', which involves acute inflammation of the tendon and its surrounding structures. Initial treatment of the latter pathology follows the same regime as any other acute musculotendinous injury, with the final rehabilitation phase being a strengthening programme in a similar fashion to that described below.

Diagnosis

Examination may reveal a degree of swelling and tenderness at the lower pole of the patella medially, whilst quadriceps contraction or eccentric loading will reproduce pain.

Ultrasound scanning (USS) or MRI (allowing imaging under the patella) are the investigations of choice, both clearly demonstrating that this condition is due to a tendonotic change within the structure, the pathology demonstrating increased matrix within the tissue, with poor collagen structure (see Fig. 10.2).

Management

Rehabilitation should include the use of an eccentric exercise programme, undertaken with the use of a decline board. This is the only proven regime that reliably produces a successful outcome, resolution of symptoms often taking up to 4 months.

Biomechanical assessment and gait analysis will assist in the overall evaluation, with orthotic correction sometimes being used to help offload the tendon. Surgical decompression may be appropriate in intractable cases. Corticosteroid injection is contraindicated because of the increased potential for rupture postinjection in tendonotic tissues.

Obliteration of the neovascularization using sclerosants, and shockwave therapy are among a number of treatments being researched at this time, in an attempt to improve the treatment of this difficult condition.

Less common causes of anterior knee pain

There are many other less common causes of anterior knee pain, for example following an injury to Hoffa's fat pad, a highly innervated structure, situated behind the patellar tendon. Inflammation may occur after a fall onto the knee on a hard surface or following repeated forced hyperextension, experienced in events such as the javelin. Tenderness can be elicited by squeezing the fat pad, with hyperextension of the knee also reproducing symptoms.

Local corticosteroid injection will produce a resolution of symptoms in those cases that fail to settle with conservative treatment, which includes taping of the superior pole of the patella to relieve the pressure on the structure.

Quadriceps tendinitis is an infrequent presentation, but may present in jumpers. Chondromalacia patellae – a term previously used erroneously to cover all causes of patellofemoral joint (PFJ) pain – is a 'roughening' of the cartilage behind the patella; it is also found in a minority of anterior knee pain sufferers. Arthroscopic retropatellar chondroplasty may be undertaken if symptoms are persistent.

Infection should always be considered in the hot, painful, swollen knee, with no clear history of trauma, as rapid joint destruction will ensue if a septic arthritis is left untreated. Aspiration will help confirm the diagnosis.

Stress fracture of the patella presents with localized patellar tenderness. The fracture can be vertical or longitudinal, with pain increasing on exercise. Isotope bone scan or MRI will confirm the diagnosis.

Other causes of knee pain

Iliotibial band (ITB) syndrome presents as tenderness above the insertion into the lateral tibial condyle, often accompanied by inflammation of the iliotibial bursa. Treatment consists of both passive and active stretching of the ITB, alongside biomechanical correction if necessary, excessive pronation often being noted. Corticosteroid injection is indicated if an associated iliotibial bursitis is unresponsive to treatment.

Medial plica syndrome is a condition where the plica, a synovial fold present over the medial femoral condyle in 90% of people, is thought to become inflamed; it is occasionally found on the lateral aspect. Examination reveals a 'click' as the finger is rolled over the structure. When inflamed it becomes increasingly painful after exercise. Corticosteroid injection or arthroscopic resection in intractable cases, are recognized treatments. The diagnosis is one of exclusion, prompting speculation about other possible underlying causes, such as inflamed retinacular tissues; as physiotherapeutic soft tissue treatments become more successful this seems to be more probable in certain cases.

Popliteus tendonitis presents in those sports that involve excessive twisting and turning. It is probably a diagnosis that is often made incorrectly, and in isolation it does not appear to be as common as perhaps previously thought. Pain is elicited on resisted internal rotation of the lower leg with the knee flexed.

In those that fail conservative rehabilitation, corticosteroid injection could be considered, undertaken parallel to the lateral meniscus, and directing the needle anteriorly from an area posterior to the LCL.

Pes anserinus bursitis is an inflammation of the bursa that lies below the common tendon formed by the insertions of the sartorius, gracilis and semi-tendinosus into the medial surface of the tibia. Pain is triggered by running and hamstring exercises, especially if tightness is present in the muscles concerned. NSAIDs and physiotherapeutic modalities are followed by a manual exercise therapy programme, with corticosteroid injection sometimes being required in resistant cases.

Referred pain can be related to hip pathology and presents with the patient having a tendency to grip the leg just above the knee. Neoplasia must be excluded, particularly in children presenting with a painful knee; osteosarcomas most commonly occur at the metaphyses of the distal femur or upper tibia.

Children and adolescents

Osteochondritis dissecans

Presentation
Osteochondritis dissecans also fits into the category of 'less common causes of anterior knee pain'. The history, usually in adolescents, is often one of discomfort in the knee, associated with swelling and occasional episodes of 'locking' if a loose body is present.

The pathology is a defect in the articular cartilage of the femoral condyle (with the loosened fragment containing subchondral bone), 80% being found on the lateral side of the medial femoral condyle. The cause is unclear, but suggestions of an underlying vascular abnormality due to repeated microtrauma have been volunteered.

Diagnosis
Examination may demonstrate a restricted range of motion with an associated effusion. Investigations, consisting of 'tunnel view' X-rays, may demonstrate a fragment lodged within the intercondylar notch. CT scan or MRI also prove useful in confirming the diagnosis.

Management
Early diagnosis is important as spontaneous healing can occur if restricted from activity early enough or arthroscopic fixation of a loose fragment may be possible, management depending on the degree of disruption. Maturation of the defect is more likely in the younger athlete.

Osteochondroses

Presentation
In the adolescent, patellar tendon problems present as one of the osteochondroses (see Chapter 12), Sinding–Larsen–Johansen (SLJ) or Osgood–Schlatter (OS) disease. The ligamentous attachment to bone, known as the apophysis in young children, is very active. Inflammation of this is an apophysitis.

The onset of symptoms is often associated with a growth spurt. Pain is noted during and following exercise, with stiffness and discomfort experienced afterwards.

Diagnosis
In SLJ syndrome, tenderness is palpated at the lower pole of the patella when relaxed, often disappearing when the tendon is put on stretch. In OS disease, discomfort is noted at the insertion of the tendon into the tibial tuberosity, with a palpable tender swelling usually being evident over the tubercle.

The diagnosis is a clinical one with further investigation not being routinely indicated.

Management
Rehabilitation should incorporate a stretching regime – tightness of the hamstrings and lower leg muscle groups being a contributory factor – combined with strengthening of the quadriceps synergists (i.e. hip extensors and ankle plantar flexors) to offload the patella.

Although it is advisable to decrease the intensity of exercise, complete rest does not need to be advocated; the previous assumption that this is a purely exercise-related condition is unfounded. The main trigger is the adolescent growth spurt and the forces it exerts on the apophysis, with excessive exercise contributing to the picture. It should be stressed to the parents that this is a self-limiting condition, although its resolution can take anything from 6 to 24 months. Whilst the diagnosis is rarely in doubt, possible injury to associated structures, such as the anterior horn of the medial or lateral meniscus, should not be forgotten (see Chapter 12).

The lower leg

Lower leg and ankle problems comprise a high proportion of the overuse injuries presenting to the sports physician. For example, shin pain accounts for up to 20% of all running injuries. The often used but inexact term 'shin splints' is unhelpful diagnostically and has tended to be used as an umbrella term for all presentations.

History, examination and further investigation help in differentiating between the common causes of shin pain, categorizing the pathologies into tenoperiosteal, muscular and bony, although this does oversimplify things somewhat as there is frequent overlap between the pathologies, as depicted in Fig. 7.9.

Medial tibial stress syndrome (MTSS)

Presentation
This is the diagnostic label given to the majority presenting within this group, although the underlying cause and pathology are unclear. Hypotheses abound, varying from a 'traction periostitis' to 'maladaptive bone remodelling'; recent studies have demonstrated a localized decrease in bone mineral density.

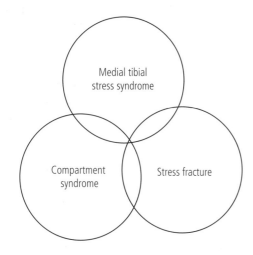

Fig. 7.9 Overlap between syndromes.

Cadaveric studies have suggested that it is soleus and flexor digitorum longus that are often found attached at the site where symptoms most frequently occur, with tibialis posterior not seemingly implicated. This may explain why effects are often compounded by significant biomechanical abnormalities.

There may be a history of a sudden change in training intensity or surface. In the initial stages discomfort commences with exercise, improving once warmed up. Symptoms then progress with the pain failing to settle during exercise.

Diagnosis
Palpation reveals tenderness and occasionally localized swelling along the medial border of the lower third of the tibia, on occasions extending more proximally.

Investigation may include plain X-rays to exclude an anterior cortical stress fracture if suspected; this is important because of the consequences if missed (see below). Radioisotope bone scan classically demonstrates a linear uptake in the delayed phase, in contrast to the focal uptake characteristic of a stress fracture or the positive early phase uptake of an acute periostitis, these findings further supporting the theories of bony involvement. MRI is being increasingly used because of its ready availability and lack of exposure to radiation. Results are more specific, with signs such as marrow oedema being common findings, indicating stress reaction with the potential of progression to stress fracture. This also clearly demonstrates the relationship between these conditions. Additional pathology may also be noted, such as the formation of a subperiosteal haematoma.

Management
Biomechanical alterations comprise either the correction of excessive pronation or increasing shock absorbency in the supinators. Physiotherapeutic modalities include manual therapy to remove soft tissue restriction and exercise therapy aimed at eccentrically strengthening the antagonists. NSAIDs are also useful in the acute presentation. Training loads and surface (e.g. track to grass) may need to be addressed.

In a number of cases symptoms become intractable. At this stage when symptoms are restricting exercise and leaving the individual with ongoing discomfort persisting between training sessions, periosteal stripping and fasciotomy is required. These tissues are often found to be scarred and thickened at surgery. Experienced surgeons will achieve up to an 80% success rate with this procedure. Return to sport following surgery, however, is gradual and controlled, as recurrence of symptoms at that stage is associated with a poor prognosis.

Stress fractures

Presentation
Tibial stress fractures are a common cause of shin pain and like MTSS tend to present with discomfort over the medial border of the tibia at the lower third/two-thirds, or less frequently the upper third/two-thirds junction. Lateral lower leg pain, with the athlete often pointing to a region approximately 5–6 cm above the lateral malleolus, is invariably indicative of a fibula stress fracture. Beware the anterior cortical stress fracture, if symptoms present away from the classically described sites, due to its tendency to progress to complete fracture with nonunion.

Runners account for almost three-quarters of all those presenting with stress fractures, with the history usually being one of pain increasing during exercise, the classically described 'crescendo pain'. Training history is important as the chances of sustaining a stress fracture increase significantly when the weekly mileage exceeds 70/week.

Pain at rest and during the night suggest more advanced pathology and should be treated with increased caution.

Diagnosis
Examination usually reveals a more localized area of swelling and tenderness than noted in MTSS, although tenderness can extend onto the anterior surface of the tibia. Biomechanical assessment may demonstrate excessive pronation, resulting in increased forces being transmitted through the bones in question. In contrast, supination is also associated with an increased incidence, as a result of the decreased shock absorbency afforded by the rigidly supinated foot.

Plain X-rays are indicated if an anterior cortical stress fracture is suspected. However, isotope bone scan will provide a result in all cases, demonstrating a focal uptake as opposed to the linear uptake noted in MTSS. As mentioned earlier, MRI is becoming increasingly popular, adequately demonstrating a stress fracture whilst also alerting the physician to the presence of a stress reaction, the possible precursor to this type of injury (see Fig. 10.5).

Management
Previous protocols have didactically suggested 6/52 rest from weight-bearing sporting activity as the norm in most cases. Return to activity should, however, be guided by symptoms (i.e pain with exercise) and signs (i.e tenderness to palpation), with activity being increased when symptom free. This regime will often help the elite sportsperson return to competition more rapidly.

Compartment syndrome

Presentation
This condition may occur within any of the compartments in the lower leg, either individually or in combination. There are four muscular compartments, divided up as the anterior, lateral, superficial posterior and deep posterior. However, only the anterior and deep posterior compartments are commonly affected, and then frequently together.

Symptoms are often triggered by a rapid increase in training load, and become more frequent as the condition develops, progressing from pain with exercise, to after pain, to rest pain (second day phenomenon). Presentation can be unilateral or bilateral, with the diagnosis being a clinical one.

Diagnosis
Symptoms are provoked on examination by undertaking resisted exercises involving the muscles in question, for example asking the athlete to heel walk to reproduce anterior compartment problems, or undertake toe raises if the posterior compartment is suspected. In established cases, 1–2 minutes of exercise will often reproduce symptoms, with tenderness then becoming evident on palpation.

Compartment pressure studies can help in confirming the diagnosis, although use of this procedure does cause some controversy, further supporting the statement that this is in the main a clinical diagnosis.

Management

A conservative approach consisting of stretching and deep tissue massage should initially be undertaken. However, most of those with significant symptoms will progress to surgery, comprising fasciotomy to decompress the compartment. In the majority this procedure is successful, with a usually speedy return to sport over the next 4–8 weeks being the expected outcome.

Calf pain

In much the same way as compartment syndrome overlaps with the other two conditions mentioned previously, to produce a diagnostic dilemma when presented with shin pain, the less common presentation of posterior compartment syndrome also requires a number of diagnoses to be considered.

Tears of the gastrocnemius are not uncommon, with the classical presentation of the middle-aged racket sports player complaining of having been 'kicked in the back of the leg' usually indicating a tear at the medial gastrocnemius-soleus junction, the so-called 'tennis calf' (see 'Tennis' in Chapter 16). Ultrasound scan, often undertaken at the time of consultation by the sports physician, will confirm the diagnosis.

Deep vein thrombosis can present in any age group, with a recent history of air travel or surgery raising suspicions. The clinical findings of a tender, swollen calf and no history of trauma are significant, with Doppler studies proving definitive.

Referred pain from the lumbosacral spine should always be a consideration, especially in insidious, intractable cases, with occasional cases of a ruptured Baker's cyst also presenting in this manner.

8 Sports injuries of the ankle and foot

Anatomy of the ankle and foot (Fig. 8.1)

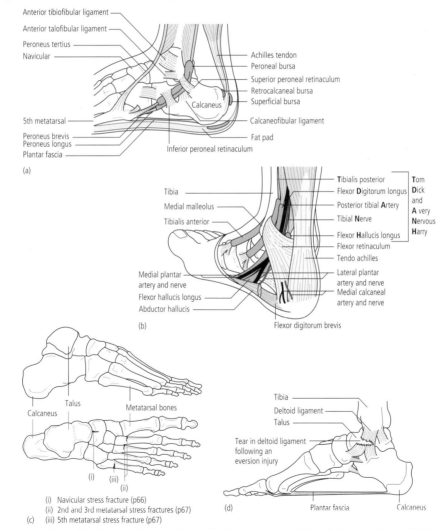

Fig. 8.1 Anatomy of the ankle: (a) lateral view of the ankle joint structures; (b) medial view of the ankle joint structures; (c) bones of the ankle and foot; (d) medial ligament structures following an eversion injury.

The ankle joint is a synovial joint formed by the articulation of the talus with the distal tibia and fibula, the latter being joined securely at this point by the syndesmosis. The prime movements are those of dorsiflexion and plantarflexion with some adduction and abduction also occurring in plantarflexion. Inversion and eversion occur at the subtalar joint. The talus spreads the joint in dorsiflexion as a result of its shape, so tightening the ligaments and increasing stability as it effectively locks itself within the ankle mortice.

Plantarflexion reverses this process, so making the joint less stable and therefore prone to injury in this position. The importance of the anatomy and mechanics of this joint become only too clear when you consider that lateral ankle sprains occur more commonly than any other sports injury.

There are a number of important ligaments around the joint, with the lateral ligaments consisting, as shown, of the anterior talofibular ligament, the calcaneofibular ligament and the posterior talofibular ligament, with frequency of injury occurring in that order. The stronger triangular deltoid ligament helps in maintaining the stability of the medial side of the ankle joint. Four ligaments and the interosseous membrane comprise the syndesmosis.

The Achilles tendon forms when the gastrocnemius and soleus combine inserting into the calcaneum.

It is surrounded by a paratenon rather than a synovial sheath. Other important structures are indicated in Fig. 8.1.

Acute injuries

Ligamentous injuries

Inversion injury ('sprained ankle')
Presentation
Inversion injury, or 'sprained ankle', occurs more commonly than any other sporting injury, most studies estimating that it accounts for about 10–15% of all injuries sustained in the sporting arena.

The history classically involves landing from a jump with the foot plantarflexed, with the athlete often being knocked off balance by a competitor. The athlete complains of immediate pain and swelling.

Diagnosis
Examination reveals tenderness over the lateral ligamentous complex, the anterior talofibular ligament (ATFL) being injured initially. More severe injuries include the calcaneofibular ligament and the posterior talofibular ligament.

Stressing the lateral joint also produces discomfort, with a positive anterior drawer test (Fig. 8.2)

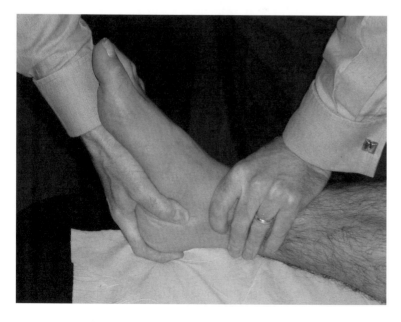

Fig. 8.2 The anterior drawer test.

confirming joint laxity as a result of a tear of the anterior talofibular ligament. Other tests often undertaken are the talar tilt to demonstrate a rupture of the calcaneofibular ligament, and the external rotation stress test, which when painful can indicate syndesmotic rupture.

X-rays should be taken if there is a suspicion of a fracture. These may demonstrate a lateral malleolar fracture or widening of the ankle mortice, which would indicate syndesmotic rupture. Failure both to examine and image the base of the fifth metatarsal is a common mistake, resulting in this fracture, a common sequela of inversion injuries, being missed.

If symptoms persist a magnetic resonance imaging (MRI) scan may help to exclude possible chondral damage to the talar dome. This may be clearly visible or be demonstrated as 'bone bruising'.

Management

The combination of rest, ice, compression and elevation (RICE) is prescribed in the acute stages (first 24 hours). Compression should be applied immediately, with sufficient pressure to restrict bleeding. Ice acts by decreasing pain and producing vasoconstriction, although this takes approximately 10 minutes to occur, supporting the need for immediate compression. The use of a cryocuff (Fig. 8.3) over the compressive strapping effectively delivers both elements.

Nonsteroidal anti-inflammatory drugs (NSAIDs) are appropriate, both decreasing inflammation and helping with analgesia. Taping is then applied over a U-shaped stirrup, both active and passive mobilization having been added after the first 24 hours. An airsplint then provides support as the athlete is guided rapidly through an aggressive regime, which has been shown to produce a speedier and more complete recovery. Supportive strapping is used once the splint is discarded. Athletes in sports such as soccer or basketball often continue to tape their ankles prophylactically, with the increase in proprioception contributing as much as the actual mechanical support provided.

Additional modes of treatment such as electrotherapy are useful in the early phase. However, it is the progression of a graded exercise programme that is the key to a rapid recovery.

Isometric exercises undertaken with increasing loads are used to strengthen the ankle, progressing to eccentric strengthening and proprioceptive retraining, often undertaken on a wobble board or trampete (Fig. 8.4).

The final phase involves the introduction of more sports-specific activities, culminating in a return to competition once full function is achieved.

A slow recovery may be associated with an anterolateral gutter syndrome or persistent posterior

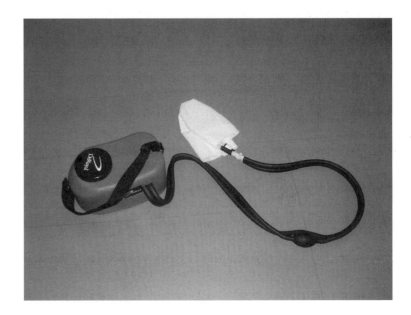

Fig. 8.3 A cryocuff.

(a)   (b)

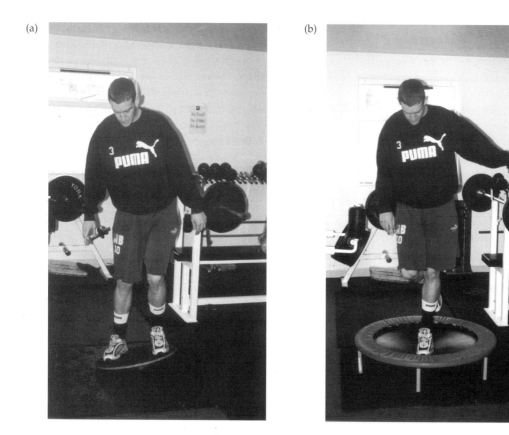

Fig. 8.4 A footballer rehabilitating on a wobble board (a) and a trampete (b).

capsulitis, with MRI useful in imaging the latter. A well-guided corticosteroid injection under ultrasound guidance often produces a cure.

More persistent symptoms may be due to complications such as a syndesmotic rupture, osteochondral fracture, or possibly peroneal subluxation. Complaints such as locking or ongoing pain during exercise indicate further investigation via arthroscopic examination, both to confirm the diagnosis and undertake the required treatment. Syndesmotic rupture is treated by the insertion of a syndesmotic screw if diagnosed early enough, whilst arthroscopic debridement and chondroplasty will accelerate the recovery of a chondral lesion.

Eversion injury and syndesmotic rupture
Presentation
Eversion injuries occur less commonly than inversion injuries, with the deltoid ligament being a stronger, more resilient structure than the lateral ligamentous complex. They comprise approximately 15% of all ankle injuries, their significance being that the increased forces required to produce this injury result in associated trauma such as medial malleolar fractures or syndesmotic rupture, classically the product of an eversion injury occurring in dorsiflexion.

Diagnosis
Clinical examination will confirm the diagnosis, with tenderness and swelling being noted over the medial ankle joint. X-rays or MRI are often requested following this injury to exclude associated fractures, chondral damage or loose bodies, the latter being a reasonably common finding.

Management
Guidelines for management are similar to those for an inversion injury once any associated damage has been excluded, although recovery times are more prolonged.

Tendon injuries

Achilles tendonitis/tendinosis

Presentation

Achilles tendonitis often occurs following a sudden increase in training intensity, for example during the pre-season football build-up or when the athlete steps up the training at the start of a track season. Training on an unaccustomed surface can also be implicated. Symptoms are initially of pain post-exercise, with a progression to pain occurring during activity. Morning stiffness is also a good indicator of severity.

Diagnosis

Examination reveals localized swelling and tenderness, usually present around 4 cm from the calcaneal insertion, a susceptible area because of its poor blood supply. In certain cases the paratenon alone is involved and this is described as paratendinitis. Presentation is different with examination revealing more generalized swelling and often palpable crepitus.

Diagnostic ultrasound is a very useful and non-invasive way of imaging the tendon. In experienced hands the differentiation between Achilles tendonitis and other causes of Achilles pain, discussed below, can be determined.

MRI can be helpful, although obviously more time consuming and expensive. However, if an experienced musculoskeletal radiologist is not available to undertake the ultrasound, it is the investigation of choice.

Management

The acute inflammatory process present in Achilles tendonitis is managed with initial rest, local treatment and NSAIDs. A gradual resumption of exercise is undertaken, slowly increasing the load on the structure. Eccentric exercises are a vital component of the rehabilitation programme and are introduced once the patient is symptom free, to increase the strength of the tendon sufficiently to allow progression to more sport-specific exercise.

There is an overlap between acute tendonitis, micro or partial tears, and the chronic condition of Achilles tendinosis, which is the cause of pain in many of the cases that present. The latter condition is a progressive infiltration by mucoid material, which replaces healthy collagen matrix leaving the tendon in a weakened state; in the worse scenario this may culminate in complete rupture of the tendon. The cause of the pain in these cases is unclear, and hypotheses vary from 'chemical mediators' to 'an increase in intratendinous pressure'.

Research appears to suggest that the only reliable way of rehabilitating these tendons is to load them eccentrically, with a level of discomfort being expected and acceptable. Weights are added as the programme progresses, with as many as two sets of 70 repetitions being undertaken twice daily (see Chapter 18).

Night splints have been used with some success and appear to decrease the amount of morning stiffness experienced, with orthotic correction sometimes being used to offload the tendon if abnormal biomechanics appear to be a contributing factor.

Recently sclerosant injections have been used to obliterate the new vessel formation (neovascularization) that accompanies the condition, and although still an experimental procedure it has yielded encouraging results.

Surgery has a place here in debriding local areas of tendinosis in an attempt to halt the process. A paratenon stripping procedure is often undertaken, removing adhesions and probably denervating the painful soft tissues around the Achilles.

Achilles tendon rupture is, as noted above, a possible associated sequela, with the athlete classically reporting that they felt as though they had been 'kicked in the calf'. Surgical repair allows the ends to be approximated and any haematoma to be removed. Rehabilitation is therefore accelerated and outcome improved.

Other tendon injuries

Tibialis posterior dysfunction often presents in athletes with excessive pronation because of the eccentric overload on the tendon. Presentation can be acute or chronic. Local treatment, strengthening and often a review of technique in combination with orthotic correction should produce a resolution of symptoms (see 'Track and field' in Chapter 16).

Peroneal tendons are also affected, with a similar management protocol being followed. In the acute case the possibility of peroneal subluxation being the cause of the symptoms should be explored, with diagnostic ultrasound being used to demonstrate the ruptured peroneal retinaculum in these cases.

Chronic injuries

Impingement syndromes

Presentation

Footballer's ankle is a condition that includes both anterior and posterior impingement syndromes. It is so called because of its frequent occurrence in soccer players. However, it may present in any sport that entails repeated plantarflexion and dorsiflexion of the ankle, posterior impingement being particularly prevalent in ballet dancers. The athlete complains of anterior or posterior ankle pain, respectively, exacerbated by the above described movements.

Diagnosis

Examination reveals discomfort on palpation over the anterior joint line or on deep palpation of the posterior capsule, with passive, forceful movements reproducing symptoms.

Anterior and posterior tibial osteophytes are usually noted on X-ray. Theories as to their origin vary from traction of the capsule, to the recurrent forceful opposition of the tibia on the talus; however, they are not osteoarthritic in origin.

Management

Conservative management is the mainstay, with soft tissue capsular inflammation often settling following corticosteroid injection. If symptoms fail to resolve, osteophytes or loose bodies may be removed arthroscopically.

Persistent cases of posterior impingement may be due to an os trigonum, a normal finding in 10% of people. This small bony remnant pinches the tissues around the posterior capsule during plantarflexion. If corticosteroid injection fails to produce a resolution of symptoms, then surgical removal should be considered.

Plantar fasciitis

Presentation

Plantar fasciitis is an inflammation of the plantar fascia, a structure that spans the medial longitudinal arch, stretching between the calcaneal tuberosity and the proximal phalanges (see Fig 8.1). Presentation tends to be in the middle-aged runner, the com-

plaint being one of pain around the medial calcaneal region. Initially the pain is most significant first thing in the morning or after sitting for a period of time, but progresses to pain with exercise.

Diagnosis

Examination confirms the origin of the pain to be the medial calcaneal insertion of the plantar fascia, often exacerbated by extending the big toe. Posterior structures such as the Achilles and calf muscles are often found to be particularly tight. The diagnosis is a clinical one with further investigation being unnecessary.

Management

Correction of biomechanical abnormalities such as excessive pronation or pes planus, either with an orthotic or a suitable shoe with support and cushioning, is undertaken in conjunction with a rehabilitation programme aimed at stretching and strengthening the involved posterior structures.

Persistent cases may require injection of long-acting corticosteroid at the point of tenderness, care being taken to avoid the calcaneal fat pad, inflammation of which should be considered as a differential diagnosis in older age groups. The use of a night splint may help in intractable cases, its function being to keep the foot in a dorsiflexed position, holding the plantar fascia on stretch.

Stress fractures (Fig. 8.1)

Stress fracture of the navicular

Presentation

The navicular stress fracture may not be the most frequent, but it is the most important stress fracture to occur in the foot. It is a diagnosis not to be missed because, as with a scaphoid fracture, incorrect management may result in nonunion and possible avascular necrosis. The presentation is one of pain, initially occurring only on exercise but progressing to pain at rest. Cases have been cited in most sports, with a predominance noted in athletics.

Diagnosis

Palpation of the navicular eliciting pain in the midline, often described as the 'N' spot, is diagnostic and should be treated as such even prior to radiological confirmation (Fig. 8.1).

MRI is now the investigation of choice, with marrow oedema (swelling within the bone) alerting suspicion. However, computed tomography (CT) will more clearly highlight a fracture if present.

Management

Immobilization in a non-weight-bearing cast for 6–8 weeks has been the norm. However, ideas have progressed and various braces are now often used with bone stimulators being trialled in an attempt to accelerate healing.

Other stress fractures

Approximately half of the stress fractures occurring in the foot are of the metatarsals, with the most common being the second metatarsal followed by the third.

Stress fracture of the fifth metatarsal appears to be an increasing occurrence in soccer, a consequence of modern footwear and increasingly hard-based football pitches. Less common, but no less important, it has a tendency to poor healing, with nonunion being an occasional complication (Fig. 8.1).

Calcaneal fractures comprise about 10% of cases, with talar stress fractures occurring infrequently and cuboid stress fractures being a relative rarity.

Other causes of foot and ankle pain

Haglund's deformity

Haglund's deformity is a prominence occurring over the posterior calcaneal region, anterior to the Achilles, and caused by friction from ill-fitting or tight footwear. The fibrous-bony swelling may become chronically inflamed, and in rare instances requires surgical removal if conservative measures fail.

Sinus tarsi syndrome

The sinus tarsi lies between the talus and calcaneum and is palpable both medially and laterally. Discomfort can develop within the sinus tarsi following overuse or trauma to the ankle, the latter often ignored or forgotten as a cause of continuing low-grade symptoms. Offloading the joint will usually produce a resolution of the condition, but persistent cases may require corticosteroid injection.

Cuboid syndrome

The anatomy of the cuboid (see Fig 8.1) leaves it prone to episodes of subluxation most commonly noted in activities such as ballet, where the midfoot is subject to vigorous dynamic forces, or hill running, in which the foot is excessively pronated. The usual presentation is of exercise-related lateral midfoot pain, with associated weakness.

Specific mobilization and manipulation often cure the problem, with the cuboid by definition being rotated rather than truly subluxed. Protective taping and support is then used during the recovery phase.

Tarsal tunnel syndrome

Tarsal tunnel syndrome presents as ankle pain radiating distally from the medial malleolus, into the region of the calcaneum and longitudinal arch and onto the plantar aspect of the foot. Symptoms occur due to compression of the posterior tibial nerve in the tarsal tunnel. A positive Tinel's test is the production of neurogenic-type pain on percussion over the area and is diagnostic.

Conservative rehabilitation including biomechanical correction usually suffices, although injection of corticosteroid may be required with surgical decompression occasionally becoming necessary in intractable cases.

Midtarsal joint injury

Midtarsal joint sprains may occur following acute trauma or in association with chronic biomechanical deficiencies, with pathology such as tarsal coalition (a fibrous union usually between calcaneus and talus or navicular) and Freiberg's disease, an infarction of the base of the third metatarsal, being considered in the younger athlete.

Morton's neuroma

This is a frequent cause of foot pain in the older athlete (usually into their forties) presenting as a gradual onset of pain between the third and fourth or fourth and fifth metatarsals, with associated paraesthesiae on the dorsum of the foot, proximal to the toes. The squeeze test and local palpation are diagnostic and help differentiate it from metatarsophalangeal (MTP) joint capsulitis, which is usually traumatic and often the consequence of worn or poorly shock-absorbing footwear ('turf toe' is a common example, occurring in the first MTP joint in soccer players).

The pathology is of a neuroma of the interdigital nerve, produced by chronic irritation, and aggravated by tight footwear. Corticosteroid injection often helps in the more acute cases, in association with attention to biomechanics and footwear, with surgical removal proving necessary in many of the more intractable cases.

Sesamoiditis

The foot contains many sesamoid bones; however, it is the medial and lateral sesamoids situated beneath the first metatarsophalangeal joint that are usually implicated.

Pain in these structures may be due to an inflammation, or 'sesamoiditis', or may be caused by a stress fracture of the sesamoid bone. Sesamoid views help delineate the pathology, with MRI also being helpful, although a bipartite sesamoid may prove difficult to differentiate from a fracture. Attention to footwear or orthotic correction help to prevent overload of the area, usually proving sufficient to produce a cure. Corticosteroid injection may be used in persistent cases, with sesamoidectomy very occasionally being required.

9 Acute and chronic injuries of the spine and sacroiliac joint

Statistics relating to the morbidity of spinal pain in the community abound and needless to say it is a common presentation. Although the athletic population may be fitter and leaner than the average, they are still susceptible to many of the factors responsible for the high prevalence of back pain in today's society.

The spine acts as a centre for all movement, protection for the central nervous system and alongside the pelvis as the scaffolding from which limb movements are initiated; this last statement is supported by research demonstrating that the transversus abdominis muscle contracts prior to movement of the upper and lower limbs. In essence the spine and pelvis create the stable base from which we can move and as a consequence instability in this area will prevent the achievement of maximal performance.

Assessment of spinal problems is often poorly taught at an undergraduate level; however, it is vital that a doctor in sports medicine develops these diagnostic skills.

History should ascertain the cause of the pain. Was there a traumatic or insidious onset? What are the aggravating and relieving factors? Is there any radiation of the pain and if so what appears to accentuate this? Has there been any weight loss? Is the pain severe? Does the pain cause waking at night?

Examination then attempts to confirm the underlying cause.

Acute causes of back pain

Severe trauma

Sports that commonly present with severe back injuries are motor sport, gymnastics, equestrian events and athletic events such as pole vault.

Traumatic injuries to the spine require expert assessment and management, and are dealt with in Chapter 2. Immobilization of the spine using a collar and spinal board requires specific training to avoid further injury to the athlete. Secure the scene, ensure safety, assess vital signs and manage appropriately; immobilize the spine and transfer to a specialized hospital unit as soon as possible.

If you are the first doctor on the scene and did not see the mechanics of the accident then the assumption must be made that a serious spinal injury has occurred until proven otherwise.

Minor or occupational trauma

Presentation of minor back trauma is common in sports such as weightlifting, rowing and hockey. These activities often result in the spine being put under load at its limits of range of movement. If the muscles are conditioned to absorb the forces in this position then structure and function is maintained, but if the muscles cannot cope with the load applied then the forces will be increasingly absorbed by the noncontractile tissues and a spinal injury may occur.

For example, a weightlifter with a poor technique may load the lumbar spine in a hyperflexed position. The result may be a compression injury to the intervertebral disc. Another example could be that of a rower with poor hip flexibility, necessitating overreaching and resulting in excessive lumbar flexion.

The ability of the spine to absorb some shock through the discs makes it more capable of coping with forces in hyperflexion as compared with hyperextension (where excessive loading may cause pathology in the facet joints and/or pars interarticularis).

As many sports people also have other occupations, contributory factors such as quality and age of mattress and work station ergonomics, if prolonged sitting is involved, must also be sought.

Tear of the annulus and the prolapsed intervertebral disc

Presentation

Injury to this area occurs as a result of abnormal compressive/shearing forces. The disc acts as a shock absorber, as well as assisting with the articulation between two vertebrae. The integrity of the disc changes with time, with degenerative change (decreased disc hydration and disc height) often occurring during the third and fourth decades of life. These changes can be accelerated in those competing in contact, collision sports, such as rugby and ice hockey. Discogenic pathology is therefore more commonly noted at an earlier stage within this group, with the alteration in the structure of the disc inevitably affecting the mechanics of the facet joints. For example, decreased disc height will result in an increased compressive force across the facet joint with axial loading leading to an increased incidence of degenerative change within the joint in later life.

An injury to the annulus often presents with the pain (especially with coughing, sneezing, prolonged sitting) being worse first thing in the morning, as a result of the disc increasing in size and volume at rest. If the protrusion becomes of significant size, the nerve roots lying posterolateral to the disc may be irritated and then compressed backwards onto the facet joints, with resulting sequelae.

Diagnosis

Examination often demonstrates an unwillingness (either conscious or subconscious) to actively flex the lumbar spine, with palpation often revealing increased tone within the paraspinal musculature. The straight leg raise test and other neurological changes are only positive if there is compression around a lumbar nerve root. Magnetic resonance imaging (MRI) is the investigation of choice.

Management

Treatment of the prolapsed intervertebral disc depends on the degree of abnormal neurology. Loss of power, tone, reflexes and/or sensation would suggest that an MRI scan is warranted (as a neurosurgical opinion may be required if there is a significant lesion producing nerve root compression). Smaller lesions may respond to manual therapy as well as exercise therapy (as the evidence suggests that bed rest makes such problems worse). For resistant cases, and those that present with significant pain and physical restriction, a caudal epidural may be of benefit. This injection (consisting of up to 20 mL of water, short-acting local anaesthetic and corticosteroid) into the sacral hiatus has been shown to reduce the inflammation and swelling around the lumbar discs and nerve roots, diminishing the pain and encouraging a far more active and speedy rehabilitation.

Having said this, some individuals suffer very few symptoms following annular tears and facet joint arthritis. This fact supports the opinion that many cases of back pain are multifactorial, with a collection of pathologies resulting in the development of symptoms.

Studies have shown that up to 50% of people who have never had significant back pain demonstrate a prolapsed disc on MRI scan, whilst other studies show that MRI scans can be completely normal in a significant percentage of those with back pain (and referred posterior leg pain).

The facet joint (acute lesion)

Presentation

The sudden overload of a facet joint (a hyperextension manoeuvre combined with rotation and side bending towards the affected side) may produce acute pain and protective spasm. Described as torticollis in the neck and being particularly frightening when it occurs in the young, this problem can also occur in the thoracic spine, and rarely in the lumbar area.

Diagnosis

Examination notes a protective spasm on the side of the pain and specific tenderness overlying the joint. The individual will express no desire to move the neck in any direction initially.

Investigation may include an X-ray to rule out the small possibility of vertebral dislocation, subluxation or fracture, if there is a history of trauma.

Management

Careful manual treatment and analgesics are the first line, with manipulation sometimes being used, as soon as the neck can be mobilized in all directions without pain, to establish a normal range of movement at the affected segment.

Chronic causes of back pain

The facet joints (chronic lesion)

Presentation

These joints may become arthritic, which will result in a change of the spinal mechanics. The athlete often presents with a vague central spinal pain, radiating several centimetres away from the midline.

Diagnosis

Pain on extension of the spine suggests that the bony elements of the spine are inflamed and are the cause of pain when they are being loaded. Investigation may comprise X-ray and either a CT or MRI scan. Stress fractures of such a small joint may be best visualized with an isotope bone scan.

Management

Inflamed joints often respond well to manual therapy (to establish improved mechanics generally within this area) and injection therapy (which can be administered using radiological guidance); studies show that injections on the outside of the joint are just as effective as injections into the joint (as the synovial membrane is permeable to corticosteroid). Radiological ablation of the nerve supply to the facets

may be considered whilst others attempt to achieve this end point using sclerosant injections (which include phenol) into the joints.

It should be noted that many senior athletes demonstrate facet joint arthrosis, but do not suffer from back pain. This supports the idea that the mainstay of treatment should be to improve mechanical function, alongside an exercise and conditioning programme for the supportive structures, reserving injection therapy for those resistant cases.

Stress fracture of the pars interarticularis (spondylolysis)

This injury (see Fig. 9.1) often occurs in sports that involve a degree of hyperextension such as cricket and gymnastics. For more detail on this pathology, see 'Cricket' in Chapter 16.

Spondylolisthesis

Congenital or acquired defects at the pars interarticularis may lead to a degree of spondylolisthesis. One vertebra may move forwards/backwards on another to a varying degree (measurable on a lateral X-ray). This apparent instability is not uncommon in sport and many cases are found incidentally (with the athlete never reporting any problem or pain). Providing the athlete is not inappropriately loading the spine (with poor technique) then the spinal and abdominal muscles should be more than capable of providing the stability that is required to perform sport at any level.

Only the most severe of spondylolistheses may prove problematic to the fit individual. In such cases a surgical opinion should be sought. The pros and cons of reconstructive surgery and the probability of the individual being able to continue to perform at their required level, should be discussed in detail.

Hypermobility

Presentation

The presentation of hypermobility may be very similar to that of hypomobility, hence the importance of good musculoskeletal examination. The symptoms are of a vague discomfort with a sense of muscular tension on and around the area of hypermobility (as a result of the constant low-grade tension of the local contractile tissues attempting to stabilize the area).

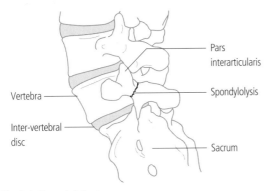

Fig. 9.1 Spondylolysis.

Diagnosis

During the examination of both active and passive movements of the spine, areas of hypermobility will be revealed to those practitioners who are accustomed to assessing the small movements that take place between the vertebrae.

The bony contours of the spine provide some stability in the neutral position. However, it is the soft tissues (especially the contractile tissues) that provide the essential stability during exercise. It has been shown that the intrinsic muscles of the spine, in particular transversus abdominis and multifidus, are in a high state of activity when the body is at rest (standing or sitting still, for example). They are constantly working as fine adjustors and stabilizers, especially before the initiation of movement.

Management

In the exercising population therefore, such instability does not become an issue until an injury has occurred elsewhere in the body (e.g. an adductor tear) and the 'stability' of the spine and pelvis are momentarily in a state of imbalance. In such cases extra diligence with this aspect of rehabilitation/self-management should suffice.

In the less fit population, areas of instability can be more problematic. Whilst rehabilitation and exercise therapy are the cornerstones to a successful resolution of symptoms, the medical profession may intervene with external support (collars and 'back supports' should be used with reluctance and for the minimum of time possible, i.e. hours not weeks). Prolotherapy to 'tighten up' the ligaments around the spine has been used with success in resistant cases.

Manipulation is contraindicated and should be reserved for areas of the spine that are not moving as much as they should be.

Hypomobility

Presentation

Hypomobility often presents with a vague area of discomfort at the site (and radiating from this site) of a restricted spinal segment (i.e. the junction between two vertebrae).

Diagnosis

Areas of restriction in the spine can be detected by careful examination. Learning to use palpation and passive movements to achieve this requires time and patience, with the movements of one vertebra upon another being subtle. This ability is essential when diagnosing a mechanical problem that requires manipulation. A facilitated segment (a predominantly osteopathic term) is an area of decreased movement and increased muscle tone, in addition to tenderness associated with an alteration of skin turgor and texture in the overlying area. Electromyography also demonstrates areas of increased activity in these mechanically deficient areas. These segments respond well to manipulation.

Management

The mainstay of treatment of lack of movement between two vertebrae is manual therapy (massage, soft tissue mobilization, reinforced articulation of the vertebrae, and muscle energy techniques, to name a few) building up to manipulation.

How does manipulation work? This has not been scientifically established because of the difficulty in evaluating subtle (functional and neurophysiological) changes within the musculoskeletal system. There are plenty of anecdotal opinions and one may conclude that manipulation is purely restoring normal function/movement of the spine, thus allowing the neighbouring tissues to return to a normal state.

There are several contraindications to manipulation of the spine, with one being manipulation of the spine under anaesthetic, fortunately outlawed in the 1980s. The author remembers many an unfortunate soul who had been 'crunched' by an orthopaedic surgeon, waking from the anaesthetic in severe pain. Further examples are the unfused spine (adolescent), infection, tumour and metabolic bone disease. Manipulation should be carried out by someone with appropriate training (in the author's opinion this should be a chiropractor, osteopath or physiotherapist/physician trained in the art of manipulation). Restoration of normal mechanics has been shown to decrease pain and allow the further steps of functional rehabilitation to take place.

The sacroiliac joint

This joint plays a key role in the stability of the pelvic ring. It is also an important shock absorber, as demonstrated by the thickness of the hyaline cartilage on the ilium and the design of the sacrum acting as a cornerstone (wedging the spine into the pelvis). The movement of the joint is subtle and difficult to assess, but appreciation of this movement is important.

Various pathologies may occur within this joint, such as degenerative change or an inflammatory arthropathy (in a similar manner to any other joints in the body). However, this chapter will concentrate on the pathology that is most relevant in sports medicine practice, which is that of dysfunction.

Sacroiliac joint dysfunction

Presentation

Distinguishing between problems of the sacroiliac joint (SIJ) and lumbar spine should be straightforward. The history may be one of injury to the joint following acute trauma (such as falling off a horse or falling on a ski slope), as a result of repetitive trauma (such as the strike leg when throwing a javelin) or as a delayed secondary phenomenon following trauma to the contractile tissues that act around the innominate, for example, following an adductor muscle tear. The discomfort is often mild to moderate; in other words it is one of those pains that the athlete can 'put up with'. The pain is often unilateral with a varied referral pattern (most commonly the anterior thigh but may occur anywhere in the lower limb). The athlete often points directly over the SIJ (despite no anatomical knowledge). Pain when rolling over in bed and local discomfort when balancing and then hopping onto the affected leg are common complaints.

Diagnosis

Examination of the sacroiliac joint consists of a barrage of tests (most of which demonstrate good intra-tester reliability but poor inter-tester reliability). Asymmetry may be present and this can be detected by palpating the anatomical landmarks of the pelvis, especially the anterior superior iliac spine (ASIS) and posterior superior iliac spine (PSIS), comparing the right and left side when sitting, standing and moving.

Tenderness over the sacroiliac joint, alongside pain with anterior/posterior movement and compression of the joint, will confirm or refute the diagnosis that has been suggested in the history. PA (posterior to anterior) passive mobilization will detect an increased or decreased movement on the affected side. Combining these findings with the symptoms complained of in the history should clearly differentiate this problem from that of disorders of the lumbar spine.

Investigations do not contribute greatly to the diagnosis, unless one suspects pathology such as osteoarthritis (X-rays and a CT scan will pick this up including any osteophytic changes), an inflammatory arthropathy or stress fracture (isotope bone scan or MRI scan depending on the preference of the radiologist).

Management

Treatment has to address the cause (if known). Hypomobility can be treated with careful manipulation in skilled hands, although as this joint is not covered by supportive muscular structures, overmanipulation should be avoided. Once manipulation has been performed, then an exercise therapy programme (rehabilitation/stabilization work) and general fitness should be worked upon. An abnormally rotated innominate (anterior rotation, for example, would result in a lower ASIS and a relatively higher PSIS on the affected side) may 'fall back' into this position following manipulation and exercise, and so reassessment with further manipulation if necessary is important, especially with chronic lesions.

Hypermobility can be addressed using exercise therapy and pelvic stability work. A sacroiliac joint belt or taping are often useful adjuncts, as are sclerosant/prolotherapy injections applied to the posterior aspect of the joint. Hypermobile joints occur during pregnancy and in those athletes with ligamentous laxity. During and following pregnancy this problem should be addressed early, with manual correction and should not be accepted as a 'side effect' of being pregnant. On returning to sport, the belt and taping can help produce an extra 'squeeze' to keep the joint compressed.

10 Radiological investigations in sport

Introduction

Imaging of the injured athlete, whether at recreational or (semi)professional level, cannot be used as a separate entity. It requires detailed discussion between the referring sports physician and the radiologist carrying out the investigation. This is not only essential to allow proper interpretation of the images, but it is the starting point of the imaging pathway, as the choice of investigations is often difficult. One has to remember that the correct choice of imaging modality (and within the modality even the techniques applied) is an important part of the diagnostic process.

Imaging has evolved from the simple yet groundbreaking X-ray of W.G. Roentgen in 1896, to an increasingly dynamic list of investigations. These investigations range from those that require ionizing radiation (plain films, computed tomography, bone scintigraphy) to those that use alternative methods (ultrasonography, magnetic resonance imaging), with increasingly sophisticated machinery allowing high-resolution ultrasonography (including blood flow assessment) in addition to functional and dynamic MRI. Such a wealth of imaging options only strengthens the initial statement that 'effective communication is essential if the use of imaging is to be maximized in the injured sports person'.

Imaging modalities

Plain radiography

Plain radiographs are obtained by placing the object of interest between an X-ray source and a photographic plate. The tissues have different X-ray absorption rates, hence the variable contrast demonstrated in the X-ray film. Although more recently, films are being replaced by digital capture equipment, the principle has remained unchanged for over 100 years.

Plain radiographs are highly suited for the investigation of bony pathology – fractures and dislocations (Fig. 10.1a) or congenital anomalies (e.g. coalition) – but poorly suited for use in soft tissue injuries. Furthermore, one has to remember that in plain radiographs three-dimensional (3D) information is completely lost necessitating the request of multiple views in most circumstances, with true 3D depiction never being achieved.

Fluoroscopy is a technique that uses plain radiographs but in a continuous fashion. Thus, one can evaluate moving structures and the integrity of joints at rest and during stress (e.g. to assess carpal instability). Traditionally, iodinated contrast would be injected under fluoroscopy to obtain images of intra-articular structures. This technique has now largely been replaced by CT or MR arthrography, although fluoroscopy is still used to guide needle placement.

Computed tomography (CT)

Computed tomography was developed in the 1970s, and is also based on X-ray technology, using a rotating X-ray source and resulting in multiple projections. This results in increased 3D information when compared with plain radiography (Fig. 10.1b). Further developments in CT ('multislice CT') now offer 3D reconstruction, which is particularly useful when planning a complex reconstruction in multifragment fractures, and for assessing structures such as the hip, tibial plateau and ankle.

(a)

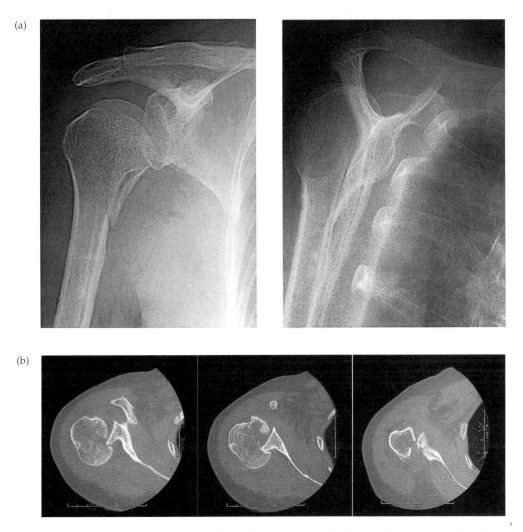

(b)

Fig. 10.1 Plain X-ray films. (a) Posterior shoulder dislocation in a rugby player (AP view). Notice how the shoulder appears almost normal, but there is subtle overlap of the humeral head with the glenoid. (b) Y-view of the shoulder, which demonstrates that the humeral head is posteriorly positioned. CT scan in the same patient demonstrates both the dislocation and multiple fragments of the humeral head.

Bone scintigraphy

Bone scintigraphy relies on the injection of radio-active compounds into the body (99m-technetium-methylene diphosphonic acid complex is most commonly employed). The radioactive tracer accumulates at areas of osteoclastic activity, thus demonstrating active bone turnover. It is a highly sensitive method for demonstration of (stress) fractures, and the use of single photon emission computed tomography (SPECT) allows for 3D visualization of the area under investigation, especially useful when assessing the carpal joints, tibia or looking for spinal pathology such as a spondylolysis. CT and MRI are, however, becoming increasingly competitive and with better specificity as well as excellent sensitivity being shown, are beginning to supersede this as a form of investigation.

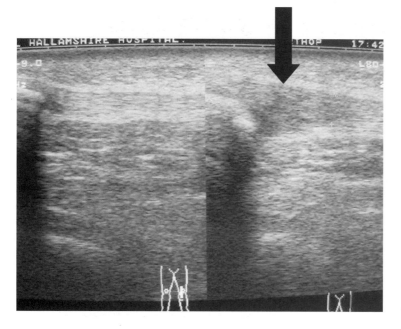

Fig. 10.2 Ultrasound of knee: patellar tendonosis of the right knee in a recreational rugby player. The left knee is normal (inferior pole of patella on left of screen), whereas the right knee demonstrates extensive thickening and low echogenicity due to granulation tissue and disruption of normally dense collagen fibres.

Ultrasonography (US)

Ultrasonography has advantages of low cost, easy access and dynamic assessment, which are set against its increased operator dependence when compared with most other techniques. Sound waves of between 2 and 12 MHz are transmitted into the tissues, and the reflections are recorded and visualized as an image on screen. The reflection of the sound beam is dependent on both the surface and nature of the tissue (Fig. 10.2).

Recent developments in US, such as colour Doppler imaging for assessment of blood flow and the introduction of so-called tissue harmonic imaging, have resulted in a renewed interest in this technology. Hand-held devices have entered the arsenal, enabling 'track-side' US to be performed, whilst also providing immediate access in the sports physician's clinic. These devices should, however, only be used with adequate training and one should be aware of their limitations (especially when examining deep structures).

Magnetic resonance imaging (MRI)

MRI uses a combination of radio waves and a strong magnetic field to produce its images. Most MR systems are 1.5 T magnets with horizontal positioning

of the patient, but open systems, the use of loading rigs and more recently the development of vertical systems will further increase their (already huge) impact on medical imaging. This is particularly true when suspecting internal joint derangement. An example in the knee joint is given in Fig. 10.3.

Acute injuries

Fractures/dislocations

Fractures and dislocations are extremely common, especially in contact sports. Of particular interest are fractures involving the spine, as incorrect diagnosis carries the potential risk of spinal cord damage. Most fractures will be demonstrated using plain radiographs, although CT may be required for more detailed assessment of more complex injuries (Fig. 10.1b). MRI is often required in spinal fractures, especially if spinal cord or nerve damage is suspected.

A small group of fractures may be imaged using bone scintigraphy, for example, suspected carpal bone fractures, which may be immobilized for a minimum of 72 hours, at which time bone scintigraphy can help to confirm or exclude the presence of a fracture. As previously noted this technique is (a)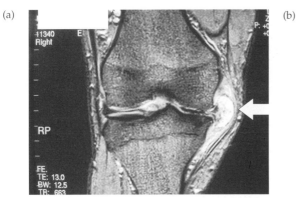

(b)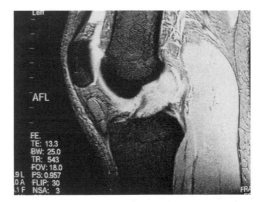

(c)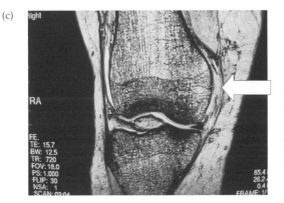

Fig. 10.3 MRI of knee. (a) Medial meniscal tear and meniscal cyst in a football player. (b) Acute anterior and posterior cruciate ligament tear in a rugby player. Notice joint effusion and 'free floating' anterior cruciate ligament and absence of posterior cruciate ligament. The posterior capsule is also disrupted with fluid outside the joint. (c) Medial collateral ligament tear in a football player (thickening and fluid seen with disrupted ligament fibres).

being increasingly replaced by MRI and/or CT, due to their ready availability.

Muscle injuries

Most muscle injuries can be adequately visualized using ultrasonography, with fibre disruption or the identification of a haematoma helping to grade the severity of injury. Ultrasonography is also useful in following the healing of muscle injuries. One of the complications, myositis ossificans, is most easily detected by ultrasonography, which tends to demonstrate calcification earlier than radiography or CT, with MRI being relatively insensitive in this instance.

More complex muscular injuries or those associated with injury to other structures are best imaged using MRI (Fig. 10.4), although, for example, when associated with bony pathology, as is often found in the groin, additional information offered from ultrasound investigation can be complementary.

Tendon injuries

Most tendons are best imaged using ultrasound as the first line of investigation, as are simple injuries to the rotator cuff. Dynamic investigation is also possible, allowing, for instance, a subluxing tendon to be visualized following retinacular disruption.

MRI is probably more pertinent when dealing with complex injuries around joints and in the pelvis and shoulder, particularly if injury to other structures is suspected.

Ligament injuries

Ultrasound can be used to evaluate ligamentous injuries in superficial locations such as the collateral knee ligaments, ankle ligaments and in the wrist. Intra-articular ligamentous injury, often associated with other pathology, is better visualized using MRI (Fig. 10.3).

(a)

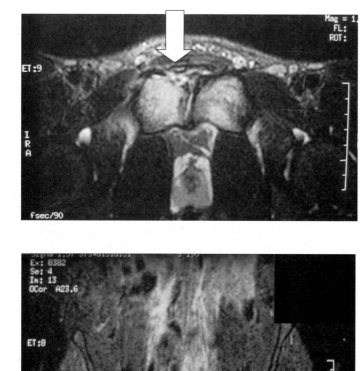

(b)

Fig. 10.4 MRI of groin. (a) Symphysitis pubis with gracilis avulsion in a gymnast. Notice the high signal within the symphysis and some high signal anterior to the right os pubis at the site of gracilis insertion on this T2-weighted axial image. (b) Adductor longus tear with a stress response in the symphysis at the same side in a sprinter (T2-weighted coronal image).

Internal joint derangement

Internal joint derangement, most commonly affecting the shoulder, hip and knee, is once again best imaged using MRI.

MR arthrography will clearly delineate glenoid labral damage, a technique involving the injection of diluted gadolinium contrast into the joint (under fluoroscopy). This technique is also of use when assessing the acetabular labrum of the hip joint.

The knee joint can be investigated without the need for contrast, and structures such as menisci and ligaments are well demonstrated (Fig. 10.3).

Chronic (overuse) injuries

The use of MRI allows stress fractures to be demonstrated as bony oedema (sometimes also referred to as microtrabecular fracture) in the early stages, indicating the potential to progress to a full-blown fracture with disruption of the cortical bone. Common sites are the tibia or the bones in the foot (e.g. navicular, metatarsals).

The diagnosis of a spondylolysis can be made using MRI in most instances (Fig. 10.5), although some discussion remains concerning the use of CT and bone scintigraphy, with many centres still quoting reverse gantry CT as the gold standard.

(a)

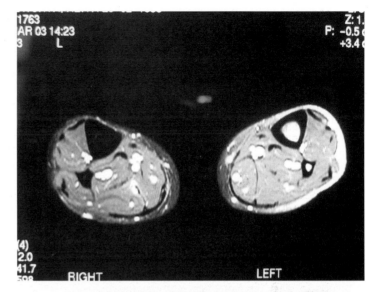

(b)

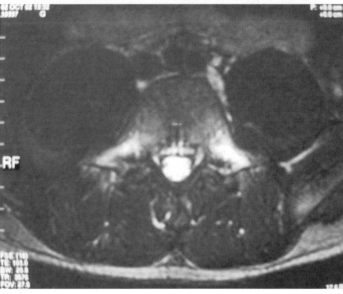

Fig. 10.5 MRI of stress fractures. (a) Tibial stress fracture in a hurdler (T2-fat saturation). There is high signal in the bone marrow of the tibia but no evidence of cortex disruption. (b) Bilateral spondylolysis in a 16-year-old football player (T2-fat saturation demonstrates high signal in both pedicles).

Osteochondritis dissecans (OCD) can be demonstrated using either CT or MRI, although the latter is generally preferred, as the extent of the bone marrow oedema is more clearly depicted.

The Achilles and patellar tendons can be well visualized using US (Fig. 10.2). Tendinosis (see Chapters 7 and 8) appears as thickening of the tendon, with loss of normal echogenicity and increased vascular signal with colour Doppler US. Paratendinitis ap-

pears as fluid within the paratenon and signifies a more acute process. MRI is also used and provides useful information relating to pathology that may exist within these structures.

Plantar fasciitis may appear as focal thickening on ultrasound, although the size of the fat pad may render US visualization difficult. MRI before and after gadolinium contrast is well suited to demonstrate this entity.

Conclusions

It is clear that noninvasive imaging techniques are more than capable of demonstrating most sports injuries. US and MRI should be the techniques of choice, with US used as first-line when looking at muscles, tendons and superficial ligaments. MRI is ideally suited for the investigation of complex body areas (shoulder, pelvis/hip), spine and large synovial joints. Stress or occult fractures may still require bone scintigraphy or CT, but MRI is equally sensitive in most clinical situations.

As stated at the outset, imaging cannot replace a good clinical history and examination. The interaction between sports physician and radiologist is crucial for the diagnosis and management of the athlete. The sports physician is actively encouraged to be present when the radiologist performs the diagnostic test, as this communication often helps with interpretation of the findings.

Finally, this chapter provides only a brief synopsis of this subject, but hopefully one that will awaken the reader's interest.

Further reading

Anderson J, Steinweg J, Read J. *Atlas of Imaging in Sports Medicine*. Sydney, McGraw-Hill, 1998.

Bojanic I, Pecina M. *Overuse Injuries of the Musculoskeletal System*. Boca Raton, FL, CRC Press, 2003.

Grainer and Allison's Textbook of Diagnostic Radiology. London, Churchill Livingstone, 2001.

Halpern B, Herring SA, Altchek D, Herzog R. *Imaging in Musculoskeletal and Sports Medicine*. Boston, Blackwell Science, 1997.

Masciocchi C (ed.). *Radiological Imaging of Sports Injuries*. Berlin, Springer Verlag, 1997.

Miller T, Finzel K. *Musculoskeletal Imaging*. New York, McGraw-Hill, 2000.

Stoller DW. *Magnetic Resonance Imaging in Orthopaedics and Sports Medicine*. Philadelphia, Lippincott-Raven, 1997.

Van Holsbeeck MT, Introcaso HT. *Musculoskeletal Ultrasound*. St Louis, CV Mosby, 2001.

11 The athlete's heart

Most sports physicians understand the risks of competitive sport. At all levels and ages sport is associated with risk, risk of injury or more dramatically risk of death. The sudden death of a young athlete is a tragedy inevitably associated with shock, grief and in some cases anger. How and why do young apparently healthy athletes suddenly die? Are their deaths preventable?

The term athletic heart describes the cardiovascular changes, including cardiac enlargement, that occur in response to physical exercise, changes considered physiological but changes that may be associated with risk. The challenge for sports physicians is to differentiate between physiological and pathological change and identify cardiac conditions amenable to treatment from those that lead to withdrawal from competitive sport.

What is the cause of the problem?

Physiology

Regular physical training leads to cardiovascular adaptation with both structural and functional changes that include an increase in left ventricular cavity size, wall thickness and left ventricular mass. Different types of activity result in different patterns of hypertrophy.

Dynamic exercise, such as distance running, predominantly increases heart rate and stroke volume, leading to an increase in cardiac output. Systemic vascular resistance falls but overall there is a slight rise in blood pressure – the load on the heart is predominantly that of volume. These haemodynamic changes can eventually lead to eccentric left ventricular hypertrophy. Eccentric hypertrophy caused by volume loading leads to an increase in the internal dimensions of the left ventricle with a proportionate increase in wall thickness.

In static exercise, such as weightlifting, although heart rate increases there is a more pronounced rise in blood pressure – the load on the heart is predominantly that of pressure. These haemodynamic changes eventually lead to concentric left ventricular hypertrophy. Concentric hypertrophy due to pressure load leads to an increase in wall thickness but no increase in internal dimension. In practice cavity size and mass are within normal limits in most athletes and patterns of hypertrophy are often mixed, as most sports involve dynamic and static activity.

The structural changes observed in the athletic heart are usually associated with normal cardiac function when compared with non-athletes, both during exercise and at rest. Diastolic function in athletes is enhanced during exercise and sometimes at rest. This increases ventricular filling at higher heart rates when the diastolic period is reduced, potentially improving performance. Although systolic function at rest may appear reduced on echocardiography in some athletes, this is often a reflection of increased diastolic volume and metabolic efficiency. This may raise concerns regarding the presence of a cardiomyopathy, which may be excluded by an exercise study to demonstrate normal or enhanced contraction in the athletic heart.

Pathology

Left ventricular hypertrophy (LVH) in athletes is usually physiological but may occur as part of a continuum with a transition from early physiological to late pathological change. This may in part be genetically influenced, with some susceptible athletes developing a pathological training response.

Left ventricular wall thickness is the single most important defining characteristic that separates physiological from pathological left ventricular hypertrophy. Athletic training increases the intraventricular septal wall and posterior wall thickness, but the increase averages only 10–15%, representing an absolute wall thickness increase of only 1 mm. Although there are some variations in the available study data, the largest survey of elite athletes showed that only 2% develop an intraventricular septal thickness >13 mm (Table 11.1).

There is little doubt regarding the cardiovascular benefits of regular exercise; however, prolonged high-intensity training may actually increase the risk of life-threatening ventricular arrhythmias and exercise-related sudden cardiac death (SCD). In some athletes persisting LVH has been reported, despite cessation of training, and this appears to be associated with an adverse long-term prognosis. Despite this, in the vast majority of activity-related deaths, a separate cardiac abnormality is identified (Box 11.1).

Hypertrophic cardiomyopathy (HCM)

Although rare in the general population this is the commonest cause of sudden death in young athletes (up to 50%). It is transmitted as an autosomal dominant condition, but may be sporadic – however, an affected first-degree relative is identified in 60% of cases.

Symptoms of HCM include chest pain, dyspnoea, dizziness or collapse but usually affected individuals are symptom free. Clinical examination is also often normal, although there may be a mid-systolic murmur that decreases in intensity on lying down. Unfortunately patients often present for the first time with sudden cardiac death (SCD).

Hypertrophy of the heart leads to a thickened, but nondilated left ventricle with an increase in ventricular mass (Fig. 11.1). This results in diastolic dysfunction with impaired left ventricular filling, mitral regurgitation and an increase in ventricular arrhythmias. Left ventricular septal thickness is markedly increased resulting in asymmetrical hypertrophy, a pattern not usually seen in the physiological hypertrophy of the athlete's heart. These changes in the septum predispose the individual to arrhythmias and may obstruct aortic outflow, resulting in syncope and collapse. Microscopy studies reveal abnormally thickened arterioles with myocardial disarray due to a bizarre arrangement of hypertrophied cardiac muscle cells with diffuse interstitial fibrosis.

Box 11.1 Causes of sudden cardiac death in young athletes

- Hypertrophic cardiomyopathy
- Arrhythmogenic right ventricular cardiomyopathy
- Congenital coronary artery anomalies
- Premature coronary artery disease
- Wolff–Parkinson–White syndrome
- Long QT and Brugada syndrome
- Idiopathic dilated cardiomyopathy
- Myocarditis
- Marfan syndrome
- Congenital aortic stenosis
- Drug abuse

Table 11.1 Echocardiographic features of the athletic heart and hypertrophic cardiomyopathy (HCM)

	Athlete's heart	HCM
Maximal left ventricular wall thickness (mm)	<16 mm	>16 mm
LVH pattern	Concentric	ASH/variable
Left ventricular cavity size	Large	Small
Diastolic function	Normal	Impaired
Left atrial size	Normal	Dilated

ASH, asymmetrical septal hypertrophy; LVH, left ventricular hypertrophy.

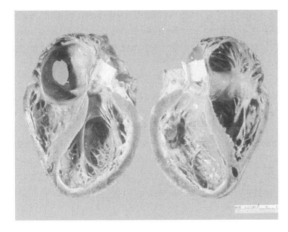

Fig. 11.1 Hypertrophic cardiomyopathy.

Coronary artery anomalies

Although very rare, these represent the second commonest cause of SCD in young athletes. The commonest variant occurs in the left main coronary artery arising from the right sinus of Valsalva. The artery originates at an acute angle, which leads to coronary flow reduction as the aorta dilates during exercise. In addition the aberrant artery courses between the aorta and pulmonary trunk, where it is prone to compression during exercise as the great vessels increase in size with the increase in cardiac output. Other anomalies include hypoplastic coronary arteries, left coronary originating from the pulmonary trunk, absent left coronary and spontaneous coronary dissection. Unfortunately most patients are asymptomatic, with over two-thirds presenting as SCD attributed to ischaemic arrhythmias.

Arrhythmogenic right ventricular cardiomyopathy (ARVC)

This is a rare but important condition associated with supraventricular and ventricular arrhythmias, leading to sudden cardiac death. The cause is unknown, but it is often familial, characterized by myocyte cell death with fatty and fibrous replacement in the right ventricular outflow tract. The right ventricle is often difficult to image with echocardiography and so cardiac MRI should be considered.

Coronary atheroma

This is extremely unusual in the young but is the commonest cause of death in athletes aged over 35. The disease is usually confined to the proximal portion of the left anterior descending artery. Premature atheroma should be considered in athletes complaining of exertional chest pain, particularly as it may be treatable with coronary artery stenting.

Marfan syndrome

This is an autosomal dominant connective tissue disorder occurring in about 1:10 000. Progressive aortic root dilatation as a result of cystic medial necrosis results in acute aortic dissection, aortic regurgitation and sudden death. The diagnosis is usually made clinically; however, genetic testing is becoming increasingly common. There is often a family history of Marfan syndrome with affected individuals typically of tall stature, with long thin limbs and fingers, long thin facies and an arm span substantially greater than height. Additional features include pectus excavatum or carinatum, hyperextensible joints, mitral valve prolapse and myopia as a result of lens dislocation. Regular echocardiographic assessment of the aortic root is recommended and vigorous activity banned once aortic dilatation is present. Because of its increased incidence in tall athletes, certain sports such as basketball and volleyball predominate.

Myocarditis

SCD due to myocarditis is often described in athletes but the exact incidence is unknown. This in part relates to the difficulties in confirming the diagnosis either clinically with myocardial biopsy, or at post mortem. Although coxsackie B virus is the commonest identified cause, a variety of pathogens have been reported. Inflammation and necrosis of the myocardium may lead to fatal ventricular arrhythmias, heart block or progressive heart failure. Progressive cardiac enlargement often occurs, with marked thinning and dilatation of both right and left ventricles.

Patients may or may not be symptomatic with a history of fever, myalgia and gastrointestinal disturbance combined with symptoms and signs of cardiac failure. 'There is [sic] little data to support the notion of vigorous exercise during a viral illness increasing the risk of myocarditis, although many physicians advise a reduction in activity when systemic symptoms of a viral infection are present.'

Disorders of conduction

Wolff–Parkinson–White (WPW) and long QT syndrome (LQTS) are among the commonest presentations in this group. WPW is due to an accessory pathway within the myocardium that permits premature excitation of ventricular muscle at rest and on exertion. It is often associated with palpitations caused by supraventricular tachycardias, and can be fatal with patients developing atrial fibrillation, ventricular fibrillation and collapse. The ECG is often abnormal (Table 11.2) although the accessory pathway can be concealed – an adenosine provocation test is required in this situation. Antiarrhythmic medication is useful in treating symptoms; however, curative radiofrequency ablation is the procedure of choice for the athlete.

The LQTS may be inherited (associated with nerve deafness) or acquired, secondary to a variety of drugs or an electrolyte imbalance. Over half of all patients will have a history of syncope, seizures or palpitations related to exertion or emotion, provoking a catecholamine surge resulting in ventricular tachycardia or fibrillation. The resting ECG is abnormal in almost all affected individuals, with prolongation of the QT interval (Table 11.2). Beta blockers and/or activity restriction are the treatments of choice, both of which are usually unacceptable to the young athlete.

Other causes

Other rare causes of sudden cardiac death are listed in Box 11.1. Many of these, particularly those associated with abnormal physical signs such as valvular or congenital heart disease, are identified in early life, some of which result in permanent exclusion from physical activity and competitive sport.

Table 11.2 Electrocardiographic changes seen in athletes and in conditions associated with sudden death

Diagnosis	ECG changes
Athletes	Sinus bradycardia, sinus arrhythmia, sinus arrest, wandering atrial pacemaker, junctional rhythm
	First-degree AV block, second-degree type I Wenckebach
	Increased P wave amplitude, increased QRS voltage (LVH criteria), incomplete right bundle branch block
	ST segment elevation/depression; tall T waves, biphasic and inverted T waves
HCM	Pathological Q waves
	ST segment flattened/depressed
	T wave inversion
	Left axis deviation
ARVC	T wave inversion in anterior leads
	Ventricular extrasystoles
	QS complexes leads v1–v3
	QRS prolongation
	Epsilon waves
WPW	Short PR interval
	Delta wave
LQTS	Prolonged QT interval
	U waves
	Repolarization abnormalities

ARVC, arrhythmogenic right ventricular cardiomyopathy; HCM, hypertrophic cardiomyopathy; IDCM, idiopathic dilated cardiomyopathy; LQTS, long QT syndrome; WPW, Wolff–Parkinson–White syndrome.

What is the scale of the problem?

The exact incidence of sudden cardiac death is unknown as much of the published data rely on individual reporting by physicians or high-profile media reports. Subtle cases at post mortem may be missed, whilst death caused by arrhythmias can be impossible to prove. Data from the USA suggest the frequency of sudden death in young athletes is low, approximately 1:200 000 student athletes per academic year. Older athletes have somewhat higher rates of exercise-related death, with rates of 1:50 000 reported in marathon runners, increasing to 1:15 000 joggers per year, the latter presumably reflecting a higher proportion of non-athletes.

Most of the identified deaths occur in young male athletes involved in high-intensity competitive sports such as football and basketball. The vast majority of deaths are in previously asymptomatic individuals and occur either during or within 1 hour of exercise. Sudden cardiac death in young female athletes is rare. Regardless of the underlying cause resuscitation is rarely successful.

How can we identify athletes at risk?

Screening for cardiovascular risk factors in the general population is relatively straightforward (family history, smoking status, cholesterol levels, blood pressure), although interventions used to effect a change may be difficult and/or their results equivocal. Screening for rare covert disease in athletes is another matter – when should we do it, how often should we do it and who should do it?

Screening young children

Screening usually begins with examination and assessment of the child at birth, with any infant found to have a murmur or symptoms and signs of cardiac disease being investigated further. Regular surveillance may then be undertaken, sometimes until the child is an adult.

Screening older children and adults

In older children and young or more elderly adults, screening for cardiovascular disease as a permit for exercise (rather than primary cardiovascular prophylaxis) is a different problem. At present there is no established facility for this, no clear consensus about how intensive the screening should be, or even a definitive decision on what should constitute a bar to physical sport. Those engaging in professional sports are likely to receive a comprehensive physical assessment, but should this not also include resting and exercise electrocardiography, or even echocardiography?

Currently different strategies exist in different countries. In the USA a noninvasive assessment is recommended, in accordance with American Heart Association specified criteria. This process is not, however, mandatory and to the concern of some, is not always undertaken by a physician. Assessment in Italy consists of history and physical examination, exercise and lung function tests, an ECG, but not routinely an echocardiogram (the investigation of choice to identify HCM, the leading cause of SCD). In the event of an incorrect diagnosis that leads to health impairment or death, the physician in Italy issuing the clearing certificate is considered liable. This despite the fact that large population studies have revealed that a standard history and physical examination rarely identifies significant cardiac disease. Within the UK there are no guidelines currently in place.

The 12-lead ECG is often used as a screening tool and certainly it is usually abnormal in patients with specific conditions such as HCM or LQTS. There are conflicting reports, however, as to its efficacy as a population-based screening tool, particularly in athletes where many different ECG patterns are recognized in physiological athlete's heart (Table 11.2). False positive rates are unacceptably high. Where there is any doubt, exercise electrocardiography can be used to distinguish normal variants from true pathology, as many of these resting abnormalities disappear on exercise in individuals without disease.

Echocardiography is essential for the diagnosis of HCM, but is unreliable in detecting other causes of abnormality in the athletic heart, such as congenital coronary arteries. Population screening using this technique is time consuming and expensive. Estimations from prevalence data in the USA suggest the need to screen 200 000 individual young athletes to identify a single individual at risk of sudden death – not to mention the large number of false positives likely, as a consequence of such an extensive programme. An echocardiography study in the UK costs approximately £200 – assuming similar prevalence data for HCM within young athletes in the UK it would cost over £40 million to identify one individual at risk. Although we can argue that the effort is worthwhile if a single life is saved, regardless of cost, who should pay for this – the state, the team or the athlete?

Echocardiography in athletes is also associated with false positive and false negative results. False positive results are due to the assignment of borderline values for left ventricular wall thickness and it can be difficult in individual athletes to determine the presence of physiological hypertrophy as opposed to pathological change. This may lead to an inappropriate ban from competitive sport. In contrast false negatives can occur, particularly if screening is undertaken during early adolescence when LVH is often absent or mild.

Management of athletes at risk

Athletes with symptoms of cardiovascular disease (breathlessness, chest pain, palpitations and syncope) should be aggressively investigated to establish the underlying cause. Ideally they should be reviewed by a cardiologist or sports physician with an interest and expertise in managing athletes with cardiac disease. Even if cardiovascular abnormalities are identified, most athletes are reluctant to adopt a sedentary lifestyle. Many are told to avoid 'strenuous' activity, but the definition of this is far from clear. The best guidelines currently available are from the 26th Bethseda Conference report (Table 11.3), which take into account the severity of the abnormality identified and the specific effects of individual sports, both in training and competition. They do not, however, allow assessment of individual risk, which is the dilemma usually faced by the sports physician in practice.

Table 11.3 Current recommendations regarding athletic participation for athletes with cardiac disease

Diagnosis	Recommendation
HCM	Excluded unless low intensity
	Older athletes may participate if favourable risk factor stratification
ARVC	Excluded
Coronary artery abnormalities	Excluded
	May participate after surgery if ETT negative
WPW	No structural disease/asymptomatic – may compete
	Symptoms – may compete if treated with ablation
LQTS	Excluded
IDCM	Excluded
Premature CAD	Low risk – allow low/moderate-intensity sport; annual review
	High risk – allow low-intensity sport; 6-monthly review
Marfan syndrome	No family history of SCD and no aortic root dilatation – low-intensity sports and 6-monthly review
	Aortic root dilated – low-intensity sports only
Myocarditis	Excluded from competitive sports for 6 months
	Return to competition if echo normal and 24-hour tape negative
Aortic stenosis	Mild aortic stenosis – may compete
	Moderate aortic stenosis – may compete in low-intensity sports
	Severe aortic stenosis – excluded
	Bicuspid aortic valve only – 6- monthly review

ARVC, arrhythmogenic right ventricular cardiomyopathy; CAD, coronary artery disease; HCM, hypertrophic cardiomyopathy; IDCM, idiopathic dilated cardiomyopathy; LQTS, long QT syndrome; SCD, sudden cardiac death; WPW, Wolff–Parkinson–White syndrome.

The enormity of the decision to recommend withdrawal from competitive sport cannot be overstated. Careful consideration must be given to the decision, ideally based on the results of several investigations, particularly where results are considered equivocal. Detraining may be required and although this is often unpopular with athletes, where there are difficulties in distinguishing pathological from physiological change, there may be no alternative. The period of detraining is fortunately short, often a matter of weeks, during which physiological hypertrophy usually regresses. Exercise testing with V_{O_2}max analysis can also be used; a V_{O_2}max >50 mL/kg/min, or >20% above predicted maximum, reliably differentiates physiological LVH from HCM.

Summary

Athletic training results in cardiovascular changes that are occasionally associated with significant risk. Sudden cardiac death is rare in young athletes, with HCM being the commonest identifiable cause. Echocardiography can identify athletes with this condition, but is unsuitable as a population screening tool. Appropriately trained sports physicians may identify athletes with underlying cardiac conditions, but a considerable challenge remains as symptoms are invariably absent.

Further reading

Johnson RJ. Sudden death during exercise: a cruel turn of events. *Postgrad Med* 1992, **92**, 195–206.

CHAPTER 12

12 Children and sport

Children in sport present a challenge to the physician who is used to dealing purely with an adult population. In various ways, children cannot be simply viewed as smaller versions of an adult. Physically, physiologically, psychologically and mechanically there are differences. Furthermore, these differences are not necessarily the same for children of the same chronological age because the spurts of growth take place over a range of years for different children.

Physiological development

Growth

To achieve full adult height children go through periods of linear growth in the skeleton occurring at the epiphyseal growth plates. The growth plate (physis) is an area of bone tissue near the ends of long bones, between the shaft of the bone (the metaphysis) and the end of the bone (the epiphysis). The growth plate regulates and helps determine the length and shape of the bone, whilst also being the last portion of the bone to ossify, leaving it vulnerable to fracture.

Linear growth is greatest in the first year of life, with a further major spurt of growth in adolescence (Fig. 12.1). In general, girls (c. 10–12) will enter the adolescent growth spurt before boys (c. 12–14) but individual variations occur. Growth is largely determined by genetic factors – tall parents generally make tall children; however, predicting height from parents' height has limitations. Using formulae will only give a 68% chance of being within 5 cm and a

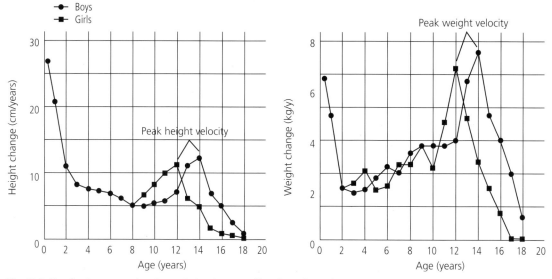

Fig. 12.1 Graphs demonstrating the variation in rates of height and weight increases during childhood and adolescence.

95% chance of being within 10 cm of the predicted height. This is because both genetic and environmental factors influence growth:

• nutrition – adequate nutrients, particularly calcium;
• illness – prolonged period of illness will limit growth;
• hormonal factors – e.g. delayed menarche;
• physical activity – stimulates bone turnover.

The growth plate is the part of the bone most vulnerable to injury, and injury may cause arrest of growth. As bone growth precedes muscle, nerve and tendon lengthening, this can lead to a reduction in flexibility, muscle imbalances and poor coordination.

As weight changes alongside linear growth, variations in body composition are noted during puberty. Under the influence of testosterone boys develop an increase in fat-free mass (FFM) as a result of muscle and bone growth, whereas girls will have higher fat mass (FM) because of the female sex hormones (Fig. 12.2).

Hormonal changes cause differences in skeletal shape (e.g. broader shoulders in males) and bone morphology, for example in the pelvis, which is often used forensically to discriminate sex (90–95% of cases).

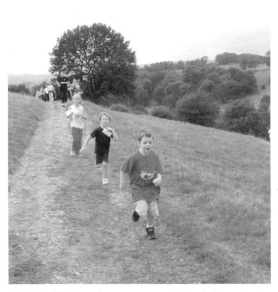

Fig. 12.3 Children demonstrate variable gait dynamics.

Exercise physiology

Children are less energy efficient than adults, with an increased energy cost per unit body weight when walking or running at comparable speeds. This partly relates to skeletal size and shape, but also to a lack of maturation of gait dynamics and efficiency of movement (Fig. 12.3).

In general they have lower absolute aerobic capacity (energy production in the presence of oxygen – endurance exercise), which gradually improves with age, with aerobic training producing little benefit in prepubescent children (Fig. 12.4). Boys demonstrate greater changes during puberty, particularly when relating aerobic capacity to body weight (mL/kg/min) with girls showing decrements as fat mass increases post-puberty.

Conversely, children demonstrate greater powers of recovery following anaerobic activity (energy production without oxygen, e.g. sprinting). Table 12.1 shows a comparison of performance between men and boys, undertaking repeated maximal sprints on a bicycle, known as the Wingate test. Body weight determines the resistance applied to the bike and the subject cycles as fast as they can for 30 seconds. Peak power and total power output are measured. The rapid recovery rates exhibited by children as

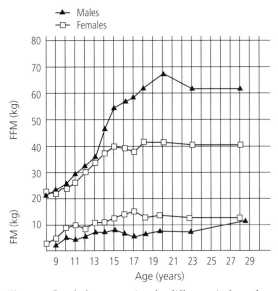

Fig. 12.2 Graph demonstrating the difference in fat and fat free mass between the sexes during puberty.

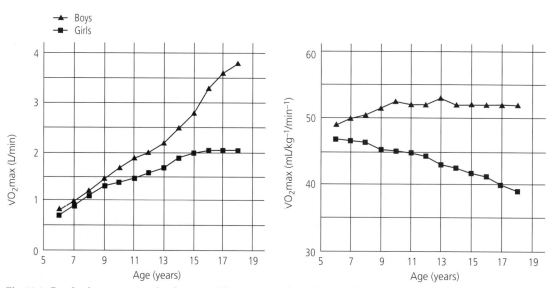

Fig. 12.4 Graphs demonstrating the change in VO$_2$max noted throughout adolescence.

documented below, may have implications for training practices.

Debate continues regarding strength training in children because of concerns over the potential damage to the growth plate. The general consensus is that the development of correct technique using low loads under supervision is important. Initially no load is used and the aim is to master the skill, with the emphasis being on control through the full range of motion. Progression is made gradually, with high repetitions and low loads building up to less than 80% of 1 Repetition Maximum (1 RM = the weight that the subject can lift only once before fatigue). Maximal intensities should only be used after age 16, and resistance training should only supplement and not replace other activities.

Exercise in the cold

Children demonstrate an increased susceptibility

when exercising in cold conditions, with a general rule being 'the younger the child, the faster the cooling rate'. A greater ratio of surface area to body mass and lower fat stores mean heat is lost more easily, with exercise in water, which has 25–30 times the thermal conductivity of air, further compounding these effects. The most at-risk child is the small, lean, ambitious individual who fails to heed the warning signs of hypothermia. Appropriate clothing should be worn and those supervising should be aware of the above mentioned risks, so as not to base suitability to continue exercising on their own perception of thermal comfort.

Exercise in the heat

Children also demonstrate a greater susceptibility to heat whilst exercising. A lower sweat rate, despite the same number of glands, results in a decreased evaporative cooling effect. Additionally, heat is produced more rapidly due to a higher metabolic rate and a greater metabolic expenditure for the same activity. Children also acclimatize more slowly, so prolonging the vulnerable period when training or competing in a hot environment. Advice on minimizing heat injury includes the following:

1 Wear clothing that covers the skin including T-shirt and wide-brimmed hat.

Table 12.1 Recovery from anaerobic exercise

	1 min	2 min	10 min
Boys	90–92%	97%	100+%
Men	72%	78%	92%

2 Avoid the sun between 11 a.m. and 3 p.m. where possible.
3 Seek natural shade.
4 Use a sunscreen with protection factor of 15 or above (25 for fair-skinned people) also offering protection against UVA.
5 Ensure regular fluid intake before, during and after exercise. Isotonic sports drinks are the most appropriate for fluid replacement, but in their absence water is clearly better than nothing at all.

The supervising adult should be aware of the potential for heat injury and ensure that children are suitably prepared for the environment. They should have adequate first aid training and be able to manage heat illness (e.g. cramps or heat syncope) should it occur. Appropriate breaks for drinks should be taken.

Obesity, physical activity and health

The incidence of childhood obesity is rising worldwide; however, there are substantial differences in prevalence between countries, with North America and Europe demonstrating higher levels. It is a depressing thought that there are now more overweight people in America than those of average-weight, so making overweight people average. In the USA the number of overweight children has doubled in the last two to three decades to a level of one child in five. As a consequence diseases such as type II diabetes are now being seen in children. The UK is not exempt, with surveys showing that energy intake has not dramatically increased but energy expenditure has fallen on average, obesity levels correlating well with the number of hours of television viewing.

Musculoskeletal injuries in the child

Despite the increasing incidence of inactivity and obesity, a significant proportion of the childhood population participate in sports or activities resulting in musculoskeletal injury. Epidemiological data on these injuries is limited, but various studies have shown that sports-related injuries can account for up to 20% of presentations to A & E in children. Acute traumatic episodes occurring in sports such as football and rugby continue to be commonplace; however, the relatively newer activities of rollerblading and skateboarding are becoming increasingly frequent causes of injury. Growth plate fractures occur twice as often in boys as in girls, most probably as a result of increased levels of participation.

Musculoskeletal injuries, as with the adult, can be divided into acute traumatic and chronic overuse injuries. However, the same mechanism of injury may result in very different pathological processes.

Acute injuries

The growth plate is held together by fibrous tissue, which although tough is not quite as strong as ligamentous tissue, making this area the 'weak link' in the growing bone. Trauma may result in plastic deformation of long bones leading to greenstick (bend) and torus (compression) fractures. However, injuries to the growth plate cause most concern, with the possibility of premature arrest of bone growth resulting in limb shortening or deformity. Any resulting angulation at the joint interface can then lead to excessive loading of the joint and premature osteoarthritis.

Any child with an acute injury, who has pain that persists or affects athletic performance or the ability to move or put pressure on a limb, should be assessed. A thorough history exploring mechanism of injury should be taken. Examination may reveal localized tenderness, swelling or deformity. Radiological studies are often required to help determine the full extent of the injury.

The two main types of acute growth plate injury occur at:
• the epiphysis – found near the end of the long bones (Fig. 12.5);
• the apophysis – found where the tendon inserts into the bone.

Epiphyseal injuries
Since the 1960s, the Salter–Harris classification has been used to categorize the majority of growth plate fractures as shown in Fig. 12.5. A more recent classification, the 'Peterson classification', adds a sixth group, in which a portion of the epiphysis, growth plate and metaphysis is missing – a less common finding following sporting injury.

In children, trauma to a joint is more likely to result in damage to the growth plate than the ligamentous structures. Growth plate fractures comprise 15–30% of all childhood fractures and are

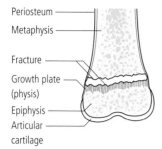

Periosteum
Metaphysis
Fracture
Growth plate
(physis)
Epiphysis
Articular
cartilage

Type I. No fracture but complete separation of epiphysis from shaft (newborn and young children)

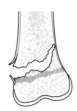

Type II. Separation from growth plate diagonally through metaphysis (MOST common presentation)

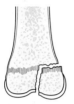

Type III. Intra-articular fracture through the epiphysis and across growth plate. Often requires surgical fixation. (Uncommon presentation)

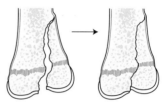

Type IV. Intra-articular fracture through epiphysis, growth plate, and metaphysis: Partial growth arrest may occur if not re-aligned as shown

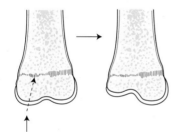

Type V. Crush force to epiphysis damaging growth plate and causing partial growth arrest as shown

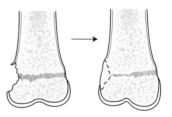

Type VI. Portion of growth plate sheared off, healing with a bony bridge as shown, with resultant angular deformity

Fig. 12.5 Classification of growth plate fractures.

most likely to occur in long bones. Being twice as common in boys, the greatest incidence is noted among 14-year-old boys and 11–12-year-old girls. The majority heal without any lasting disability; however, a number of factors influence whether long-term damage occurs:
• the severity of the injury;
• the age of the child – younger ages have more potential for problems;

• type of growth plate fracture – see classifications;
• site – e.g injuries at the knee produce the greatest risk of premature growth arrest.

Children demonstrate more rapid bone healing. The down side of this is that delay in diagnosis may mean that healing in malalignment has already commenced, whilst on the positive side, the period of immobilization required will be reduced. General rules regarding fracture management are outlined in Table 12.2.

Table 12.2 General rules regarding fracture management

Type		Treatment	Prognosis
I	Epiphysis separated from metaphysis but growth plate intact	Cast	Good
II	Most common Epiphysis, together with the growth plate, is partially separated from the metaphysis	Cast +/– reduction (occ. surgery)	Generally good
III	Rare Fracture runs completely through the epiphysis	Surgery	May result in arrested growth
IV	Fracture runs through the epiphysis, across the growth plate, and into the metaphysis	Surgery – internal fixation	Need to ensure alignment of joint surfaces to prevent OA and or arrested growth
V	Compression injury to growth plate	Surgery – internal fixation	Commonly results in arrested growth of the bone
VI	Part of the epiphysis is missing, usually through compound injury	Surgery +/– later reconstructive surgery	Arrested growth of bone almost inevitable

Osteochondroses

The term 'osteochondrosis' encompasses a number of conditions affecting the growth plate, with a variety of postulated causes. Some, for example Kohler's disease of the navicular, are thought to be avascular in origin, whilst others, for instance Osgood–Schlatter disease of the tibial tubercle, have a definite association with activity.

Three groups exist:

1 **Articular:** e.g. Perthes' disease of the hip, Kienböck's (lunate), Freiberg's (metatarsal), Panner's (capitellum – humerus), osteochondritis dissecans (medial femoral condyle – knee).

2 **Nonarticular:** i.e. traction apophysitides occurring following recurrent loading of the growth plate at tendinous attachments; e.g. Sever's disease (calcaneum), Osgood–Schlatter disease (tibial tubercle), Sinding–Larsen–Johansson (lower pole of patella) (see 'Chronic overuse injuries' below).

3 **Physeal:** e.g. Scheuermann's disease affecting the thoracic vertebral end plates, associated with juvenile-onset thoracic kyphosis. Anterior vertebral wedging may occur, with X-rays showing end-plate irregularities and Schmorl's nodes formation.

Acute apophyseal injuries

Ligament and tendon injuries occur less frequently than epiphyseal and apophyseal injuries. However, certain forces may be associated with an acute avulsion at the bone–tendon junction (apophysis). Injury may occur following a blocked kick or an explosive movement, with the most commonly affected sites listed below:

- lesser trochanter – iliopsoas;
- anterior inferior iliac spine – rectus femoris;
- anterior superior iliac spine – sartorius;
- ischial tuberosity – hamstrings;
- inferior pubic ramus – gracilis.

A classical history, with localized tenderness at the insertion and pain reproduced on stretching the relevant muscle, should raise suspicion. Tight quadriceps and hamstrings alongside a history of a recent growth spurt are common findings, all adding to the susceptibility of the bony attachment. Unless there is marked separation, surgery is not indicated and conservative treatment leads to full recovery, but this may be lengthier than a soft tissue injury. Attention to restoring full flexibility during the rehabilitation programme is imperative.

Other important acute injuries

Several other acute musculoskeletal injuries are seen in children, sometimes as a result of sporting or leisure pursuits.

Tibial spine avulsion fracture: an epiphyseal injury that is equivalent to an isolated rupture of the anterior cruciate ligament in the adult. Anterolateral instability of the knee may result. Anterior cruciate ligament and collateral ligament injuries do occur but are more common in the older adolescent.

Valgus and varus stress injuries to the knee: these may present as joint laxity. Stress X-rays may demonstrate a fracture of the growth plate of the distal femur/proximal tibia. Distal femoral physeal injuries have a higher incidence of growth discrepancy than physeal injuries elsewhere.

Meniscal injury: this is uncommon in childhood unless there is an abnormality, e.g. a discoid meniscus.

Avulsion of the tibial tubercle: this is associated with a forceful landing on a flexed knee.

Injury to the distal fibular epiphysis: this may present as a lateral ankle ligament injury.

Acute traumatic separation of the upper femoral epiphysis: this is rare but an acute exacerbation of a chronic slipped upper femoral epiphysis is not uncommon. Complications include malunion and avascular necrosis of the hip.

Chronic overuse injuries

Training has become more intense in children, and participation in sport commences at an earlier age, with talent identification programmes attempting to spot future champions, whilst wilful parents push them on to achieve success. The result can be the presentation of a variety of chronic or overuse injuries. Some are sports specific, for example the repetitive loading of the medial elbow in baseball pitching leading to damage to the medial epicondylar growth plate, known in the USA as 'Little Leaguer's elbow'.

A variety of other factors can also lead to an increased risk of injury in the child. These may be classified as intrinsic (within the body) or extrinsic (outside of the body), and are outlined in Table 12.3.

Following a growth spurt there will be changes in flexibility and coordination. A child who has grown, for example, 10 cm in a year will need time to adapt to the new muscle length and changes within his or her lever system. The motor programmes developed to perform activities will have to be revised and refined for these new parameters, with the once graceful dancer become temporarily ungainly, until the new skills are acquired. During this period, the risk of injury is greatest. The temptation may be to push on and train harder when what is required is a reduction in training load, concentrating on flexibility and skill reacquisition. Table 12.4 summarizes overuse injuries that are unique to the child athlete.

Osgood–Schlatter disease

Osgood–Schlatter disease is a traction apophysitis of the patellar tendon insertion into tibial tubercle. Repeated contraction of the quadriceps muscle pulling on the patellar tendon can cause inflammation, softening and partial separation of the cartilaginous growth plate. It generally affects:

Table 12.3 Factors leading to an increased risk of injury in the child

Intrinsic factors	Extrinsic factors
Growth (susceptibility of growth cartilage to repetitive stress, inflexibility, muscle imbalance)	Too-rapid training progression and/or inadequate rest
Inadequate conditioning	Inappropriate equipment/footwear
Anatomical malalignment	Incorrect sporting technique
Menstrual dysfunction	Uneven or hard surfaces
Psychological factors (maturity level, self-esteem)	Adult or peer pressure
Prior injury	

Table 12.4 Summary of overuse injuries unique to the child athlete

Body region	Common sport	Overuse injury
Shoulder	Tennis	Proximal humeral growth plate
Elbow	Baseball	Medial epicondylar growth plate
Wrist	Gymnastics	Wrist growth plates
Spine	Gymnastics	Stress fracture of pars interarticularis
Hip/pelvis	Athletics – track	Ischial/iliac crest growth plate
Knee	Football	Osgood–Schlatter disease/Sinding–Larsen–Johansson disease
Ankle/heel	Soccer	Sever's disease – calcaneal apophysis
Foot	Dancing	Iselin's disease – base of fifth metatarsal

- males aged 10–15 years;
- females aged 8–13 years;
- preponderantly males, with M:F ratio = 3:1.

Often bilateral, it is usually associated with a high level of activity, particularly running, jumping and kicking, and with sports such as football, basketball and gymnastics. The presentation is of pain and tenderness over the tibial tubercle, which is aggravated by activity. It is exceedingly common and is self-limiting but can persist for up to 2 years.

The diagnosis is usually based on clinical grounds – localized tenderness and swelling, tight quadriceps and a history of a recent growth spurt (probably the most relevant factor in this condition). An X-ray is not usually required but is occasionally undertaken to reassure the parent or to look for a detached ossicle in the older patient.

Management
- Modification in activity – while there is no evidence that rest accelerates the healing process, a reduction in activity will reduce pain. There is no need to rest completely unless pain prohibits it.
- Stretching – it may be associated with tight quadriceps and hamstring muscles and these should be regularly stretched.
- Ice – application of ice for 15–20 minutes after activity may reduce discomfort.
- Orthotics – sometimes there is a biomechanical problem in the foot causing excessive pronation, which causes the lower leg to internally rotate and create a shear force, which may aggravate the problem. In this case an orthotic worn in the shoe may help.

- Rarely a small fragment of bone at the tibial tuberosity may separate and if this causes persistent symptoms it may have to be excised. This can cause persistent symptoms in the more skeletally mature patient.

Sever's disease
In a similar manner to Osgood–Schlatter disease, Sever's disease affects the Achilles insertion into the calcaneum, and occurs especially in jumping/landing activities such as gymnastics. Tight gastrocnemius and soleus muscles are often an underlying cause in association with a growth spurt. (See 'Management' under 'Osgood–Schlatter disease' above for principles of treatment.)

Freiberg's disease
Freidberg's disease is an osteochondrosis affecting the metatarsal head, usually the second. Pain and tenderness on clinical examination are usually sufficient to make the diagnosis; however, an X-ray may demonstrate the progression of the disease, with advanced cases demonstrating 'flattening of the head'. Offloading the joint and reducing activity are usually sufficient to produce a cure.

Stress fractures
Excessive loading and/or inadequate recovery from training may lead to stress fractures in bone. They occur more commonly in adults, but one should be mindful that they do occur in children. The tibia is most commonly affected (as in adults). Other sites include the metatarsals (runners) and pars interarticularis (associated with repeated hyperextension

of the lumbar spine, common in gymnasts, divers and cricket bowlers). However, any of the adult sites may be involved.

X-ray will identify about 50% of stress fractures, but changes may not be evident for several weeks after symptoms present. If there is clinical suspicion despite a normal X-ray, a magnetic resonance imaging (MRI) or isotope bone scan may be required to identify the fracture. MRI has the advantage of incurring no radiation exposure, and is therefore preferred, but cost and availability may preclude it.

Treatment advice is generally to rest, with a graduated return to sport; however, some may require protective bracing, casting and occasionally surgery.

Other orthopaedic conditions

Tarsal coalition

This is the congenital fusion of tarsal bones with a bony or cartilaginous bar. Discomfort is noted with activity. The most common union is between calcaneus and talus or navicular. Orthotics may be of use, but surgery would be the treatment of choice in intractable cases.

Slipped capital femoral epiphysis

The typical presentation is of an overweight 12–15-year-old male, presenting with a limp. Referred pain to the knee is not uncommon. Examination may demonstrate that the leg is shortened and externally rotated. The condition is often bilateral.

X-ray will confirm the diagnosis and orthopaedic assessment should be urgently pursued.

Osteogenic sarcoma

Commonly affecting the lower femur and upper tibia or humerus, this aggressive malignant tumour presents in the 10–25-year age group, with males predominating. The general complaint is one of pain and swelling, which patients sometimes blame on an injury.

X-ray will confirm the diagnosis and management is urgent surgical intervention.

Osteoid osteoma

This is a benign tumour of unknown aetiology. It can occur in any bone, but in approximately two-thirds of patients the appendicular skeleton is involved. Most patients are young, with a male:female ratio of 2:1.

The classic presentation is of localized bone pain at the site of the tumour, which is worse at night and increases with activity. Dramatic relief is achieved with small doses of aspirin, which often highlights the diagnosis.

13 Women in sport

Physiological differences between the sexes

There are a number of physiological differences between men and women, which result in a potential disadvantage to women in terms of sporting performance when directly comparing the sexes. Women have a lower lean muscle mass (i.e. higher body fat) than men, affecting their power to weight ratio. Women also have, on average, a lower level of haemoglobin, affecting oxygen-carrying capacity and therefore aerobic potential. Consequently values for Vo_2max are lower in women than in men, even when differences in body composition are taken into account.

Anthropometric measurements differ, with men overall being 7–10% bigger than their female counterparts. Within this, men have a wider shoulder span, affording greater leverage and therefore greater relative upper body strength. Because of the large overlap between the male and female ranges, the difference in performance between the two sexes is only truly apparent at the elite level, where the best male athlete is likely to outperform the best female athlete in most sporting events. The best female athlete is still likely to outperform the majority of males.

Historically there have been, and still are, social barriers for women to overcome in sport, and consequently their full potential in many disciplines may be yet untapped. In the last 50 years, the women's world record as a percentage of the men's, has increased in practically all sports, and approaches over 90% in most. For example, the world record for the women's 100 m sprint is now 95% of the men's record; in 1950 it was 88.7%. It is, however, probably still not yet possible to truly gauge the physiological difference, independently of social factors (Fig. 13.1). One sport in which women do excel as a result of these differences is open water swimming, where the higher relative body fat of women aids buoyancy and protects from the effects of cold on performance.

Apart from the wider general health benefits accrued through regular exercise, there are further proven health benefits specific to women. Bone mineral density is both increased and protected through regular weight-bearing and resistance

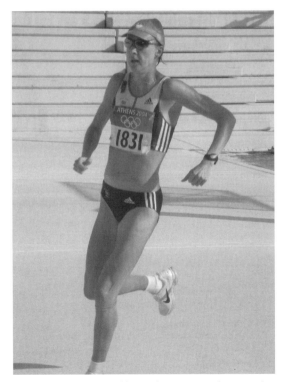

Fig. 13.1 Women's world records are approaching men's in all sports.

97

exercise, in both pre- and post-menopausal women. Studies have shown that women who exercise regularly also experience fewer unwanted premenstrual symptoms and less dysmenorrhoea. Thus, unless medically contraindicated, regular exercise should be encouraged for all women as part of a healthy lifestyle.

Menstruation

Although there is no demonstrable physiological decline in performance and no confirmed propensity to increased injury rates associated with menstruation, some women feel that they are unable to perform to their best at this time, particularly if they suffer from significant dysmenorrhoea. In the competitive athlete this can be managed through the use of the oral contraceptive pill, which can be timed to prevent withdrawal bleeds occurring during competition. The pill-free week, or inactive pills, can also be missed, with packets being taken 'back to back', so preventing any bleed at all.

NSAIDs (nonsteroidal anti-inflammatory drugs) are generally the drugs of choice for management of dysmenorrhoea (painful periods), usually in the form of mefenamic acid, because of their effect on prostaglandin activity, thought to be involved in the mechanism of this condition.

Athletic amenorrhoea

Amenorrhoea resulting from intense physical training is not uncommon in competitive female athletes. It results from disturbance of the hypothalamic-pituitary axis causing low levels of circulating oestrogen. Most presentations are in endurance sports (e.g. distance running), sports requiring a high power to weight ratio (e.g. gymnastics), where a particular body type is also considered to be aesthetically desirable, and other disciplines such as lightweight rowing, where athletes can only compete if they make a set weight. It is, however, a very rare occurrence in power athletes.

Up to 50–60% of women running 60–80 miles per week will experience menstrual irregularities (either amenorrhoea or oligomenorrhoea), this figure falling to 20% in women running only 20 miles per week. Factors predisposing to athletic amenorrhoea

include low calorie intake, low body fat and, independently, low body weight. External factors, such as high psychological stresses, either within or outside the sporting arena, can also be causative, as can other conditions, in particular, eating disorders.

Prolonged amenorrhoea predisposes the athlete to the development of lowered bone mineral density at a time in life when it should be maximized (from menarche to the mid-30s). As a consequence the likelihood of training-related stress fractures and the risk of future osteoporosis is increased, in addition to the more obvious short-term effects on fertility.

Athletic amenorrhoea is reversible, and advice should be to decrease training intensity, increase calorie intake and increase body fat/mass to the point where menstruation returns. These measures should be undertaken with care and moderation in order to maximize compliance and prevent defaulting.

The diagnosis of athletic amenorrhoea requires a clear history of secondary amenorrhoea coinciding with an increase in training volume or an exercise-related weight loss, with no other pathological cause. The clinician should investigate along the usual lines, sufficient to satisfy themselves that no other cause of amenorrhoea has been overlooked. In cases of athletic amenorrhoea of longer than 6 months' duration, management involves the use of hormonal supplementation, usually either hormone replacement therapy (HRT) or an oral contraceptive pill, and radiological estimation of bone mineral density.

The coexistence of athletic amenorrhoea, eating disorder and a low bone mineral density is commonly known as the 'female athlete triad'. Treatment should be undertaken by a specialist familiar with this type of condition, usually within a specialized multidisciplinary team. It is generally accepted that the combination of dietary strategy, training modification, hormonal manipulation and cognitive behavioural therapy alongside the management of bone pathology, if necessary, form the mainstay of treatment of this condition. Long-term follow-up and support may be required to achieve a lasting effect. The desire for sporting success is a 'carrot' that can be dangled in front of the female athlete with an eating disorder, to encourage compliance, where none can sometimes be found in a more sedentary sufferer.

Exercise and pregnancy

Although the initial anabolic effects of the hormones of pregnancy, particularly human chorionic gonadotrophin, which has similar properties to human growth hormone, can result in an early maintenance or even improvement in athletic performance, the consequent physiological changes of pregnancy, including increased body weight, shift in centre of gravity, compression of the lungs by the gravid uterus and ligamentous laxity, inevitably result in a decline in sporting activity as pregnancy progresses. It has been estimated by various studies that 50–90% of previously active women will have stopped exercising by the time they reach term. In regular runners, performance has decreased to 50% of preconception levels by the third trimester. Non-weight-bearing exercise such as swimming and cycling is tolerated more easily.

The following are absolute contraindications to exercise during pregnancy:
1 Pregnancy-induced hypertension.
2 Preterm rupture of membranes.
3 Preterm labour during the previous or current pregnancy.
4 Incompetent cervix.
5 Persistent second or third trimester bleeding.
6 Intrauterine growth retardation.

There is no evidence to suggest that continuing to exercise during a normal and straightforward pregnancy adversely affects either mother or fetus. Studies have recorded improved perinatal outcomes in mothers who undertake regular, moderate aerobic exercise through pregnancy, when compared with sedentary controls. These outcomes include shorter hospital stay, less frequent instrumental delivery, shorter duration of labour and higher infant Apgar scores. However, low birthweight has been recorded in babies born to mothers who exercised very vigorously through the pregnancy, although this decrease is characterized by lower infant body fat rather than difference in head circumference or crown rump length. The long-term significance of this, if any, is not known.

The American College of Obstetricians and Gynecologists recommends that a pregnant woman can safely exercise at the same level as in pre-pregnancy, but that training volume should not increase. Some health professionals have reservations about anaerobic exercise (e.g. weight training), particularly in those who use the Valsalva manoeuvre during strenuous lifting and abdominal muscle strengthening during pregnancy. Studies have not been performed on these types of exercise and no reliable guidance can therefore be provided.

Care should be taken when advising previously sedentary women who decide to take up exercise for the first time during pregnancy. A regular and gradual routine of initially very gentle exercise should be undertaken, ideally under the supervision of an appropriately qualified instructor or through attendance at an exercise class specifically for pregnant women.

Risks to mother and fetus are minimized by bearing in mind the following:
1 There is an established link between increased maternal core temperature and teratogenesis. Exercise in hot environmental conditions should be discouraged and hydration must be conscientiously maintained by frequent consumption of water, isotonic sports drink or other appropriate fluids. Exercise in water helps to control core temperature.
2 Dietary energy intake must increase by approximately 300 kcal per day to maintain a normal pregnancy. This must be taken into account during prolonged periods of exercise, particularly as the pregnant woman is physiologically more vulnerable to hypoglycaemia. A high-carbohydrate meal or snack should be taken 2–3 hours before exercise to ensure adequate muscle glycogen stores and blood glucose levels.
3 As pregnancy progresses there is increased vulnerability to direct trauma to the abdomen, both because the uterus is larger and more prominent and because the resulting change in centre of gravity can increase the tendency to overbalance and fall. Uneven surfaces, stray rackets and even kicking feet in a busy swimming pool present potential risks worth considering. Contact sports should be stopped once the fundus has risen above the pelvic brim.
4 Although ligamentous laxity occurs late in pregnancy and therefore is unlikely to be the limiting factor to exercise, care should be taken not to overstretch joints during flexibility exercises. Postnatally the laxity persists for some weeks, levels of progesterone only returning to normal at around

12 weeks post partum. A return to contact sport should therefore be delayed until this time.

Infertility in the female athlete

Clearly female athletes are as vulnerable as any other women to the many causes of infertility. Additionally athletic amenorrhoea is a possible cause of infertility, presenting in endurance athletes or where low body weight and/or body fat exist. Cessation of training, in some cases necessary for up to 6 months, should result in a return of menses, and if this is not the case, further investigation is necessary.

In power athletes, the possibility that anabolic steroids are being used should be considered (in the potential father too, if he is also a power/strength athlete). Although this is widely perceived to be a phenomenon exclusive to elite and professional athletes, studies have shown higher than expected levels of anabolic steroid abuse in recreational and college athletes.

Intersex conditions can, depending on the type, result in greater than usual athletic prowess coexisting with an anatomical and/or hormonal inability to conceive in a woman. This must be dealt with sensitively and with the greatest of discretion with regard to those in the public eye and with professional reputations to protect.

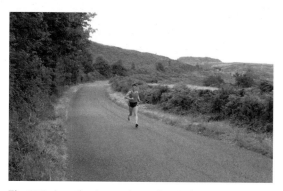

Fig. 13.2 A mother's exercise regime is the greatest determinant of a family's exercise habits.

Wider social implications

The multiple health benefits of regular exercise are indisputable and widely recognized, yet two-thirds of the UK population remain sedentary. It is known that those who exercise in childhood and adolescence are more likely to continue to do so through adulthood.

Studies show that the greatest determinant of whether a family exercises regularly or not is whether the mother engages in regular exercise herself (Fig. 13.2). It therefore behoves all healthcare professionals to encourage women, where possible, to engage in regular exercise for their own health and for the wider health of the population

14 The veteran athlete

Introduction

The term 'veteran athlete' is broad. In many competitive sports, participants can be classified as veterans in their late twenties. For the purposes of this chapter, we look at those exercising into older age. It is important to remember that age-related physiological changes occur from the fourth decade and that a vast continuum of physical activity exists for this age group, from the elite masters athlete, to those wishing to remain independently active.

The age of 65 is an age milestone used in recommendations for exercise in the older population. In the UK, population growth is fastest in those over 65 years. In 2000, a fifth of the population was said to be over 60. In 2030 it is predicted that this proportion will rise to a third.

Two key issues arise from this population growth, which have an impact on sport and exercise medicine. Firstly, with increasing numbers living longer, more will remain physically active, increasing demand for sports medicine services. Secondly, this section of the population typically has high health and social care demands, placing strain on budgets for these services. However, an active and healthy ageing population may ameliorate these costs and thus we should promote physical activity to our patients. Population studies have consistently shown that better health habits lead to longer, healthier lives with the onset of disability compressed into fewer years at the end of life.

The physiology of ageing

All systems in our body undergo changes as we age. Some of the key systems are outlined below.

Cardiovascular system

Changes to the cardiovascular system have been extensively studied, although information is conflicting due to the difficulty in distinguishing the effects of ageing from those of inactivity or disease. Maximal oxygen consumption (Vo_2max) is said to be the most reliable indicator of cardiovascular fitness. Studies show that beyond the age of 35 years Vo_2max starts to decline, by approximately 1% per year. This only becomes significant in individuals taking part in sports requiring near maximal oxygen consumption. It is also known that the more active an individual, the slower the rate of decline. Studies comparing exercisers to nonexercisers found a 13% decrease in Vo_2max in the exercisers over a 23-year period compared with 41% in the nonexercisers. The combination of decreased stroke volume and heart rate (even at high exercise intensities) leads to decreased cardiac output, resulting in less oxygen-rich blood arriving at the working tissues. The heart also becomes less compliant through small changes in collagen, elastin and reticulin contents. This is insignificant at rest, but during exercise it may reduce ventricular filling and thus cardiac output.

Atherosclerosis, to varying degrees, is almost universally present in ageing adults, leading to narrowing of vessels and a reduction of blood supply (and thus performance) to the muscles.

Studies in the elderly have shown that small increases, through modest exercise training, in Vo_2max may make the difference between living independently or requiring institutionalized care.

Respiratory system

Many factors influence respiratory function. Age-related changes include an increase in respiratory effort during physical activity, with older participants feeling more out of breath whilst undertaking activities that they would previously have found easy. Lung compliance and thoracic wall mobility decrease with age, both intrinsically and as a result of factors such as exposure to pollution and incidence of respiratory disease.

These changes lead to decreased inspiratory capacity and forced expiratory volume, decreased total lung capacity and tidal volume, increased residual lung volume and reduced inspiratory airflow. To compensate the older athlete increases respiratory rate when exercising, rather than tidal volume.

Musculoskeletal system

Most studies have looked at bone changes because of the morbidity and mortality associated with osteoporosis. Osteoporosis is categorized into type 1, comprising women affected due to postmenopausal loss of oestrogen, and type 2, affecting both sexes as a result of ageing, the latter being compounded in those leading a sedentary lifestyle. Osteoporotic fractures, usually affecting vertebrae and hips, are a complication associated with a high morbidity and mortality, most frequently seen in women and often occurring following only minor trauma.

Muscular size and strength decreases with age, especially in those over 60 years. The reduction in muscle mass is principally due to loss of muscle fibres, but also represents a change in ratio of type 1 to type 2 fibres (the change being an increase in type 2).

Alterations occur within the collagen of ligaments and tendons, decreasing these structures' compliance and healing capacity whilst increasing their vulnerability to injury. Bony resorption occurs at the site of tendon and ligament insertions, therefore requiring less force to produce a complete disruption or avulsion fracture. One should note that all these age-related changes are reversible with regular exercise.

Similarly the compliance of articular cartilage decreases as a result of alteration of cross-linkage stabilization of the collagen, producing brittle, less resilient cartilage. Inactivity compounds these changes, leading to atrophy.

Box 14.1 Summary of health benefits of physical activity

Cardiovascular risk ↓

Blood pressure ↓
Improved lipid profile
Improved glucose tolerance
Body weight ↓

Falls ↓

Sarcopenia ↓
Mobility ↑
Muscle strength ↑
Coordination ↑

Miscellaneous

Cognitive function ↑
Feeling of well-being ↑

Benefits of exercise

The benefits of exercise are well established and have a good evidence base. These are summarized in Box 14.1. Importantly, physical activity needs to be regular and sustained, as most benefits are lost over time on cessation of exercise.

Cardiovascular

There is a large body of evidence, derived from population studies, indicating that a number of cardiovascular risk factors can be reduced by exercise.

Hypertension
Endurance exercise training has been shown to lower systolic and diastolic blood pressure in mild hypertensives (by 5–11 mmHg). Light to moderate exercise (walking) is known to be effective in lowering blood pressure in older hypertensives.

Hypercholesterolaemia
Plasma lipid profiles improve with exercise; however, it is unclear if these changes are independent of changes in body composition (fat stores). Those who are generally more active are known to have mod-

estly better lipid profiles when compared with sedentary individuals. High-density lipoprotein (HDL) levels increase whilst very-low-density lipoprotein (VLDL) and triglyceride (TG) levels decrease. These changes are thought to be due to the increased activity of lipoprotein lipase and prolonged HDL survival.

Glucose tolerance

Regular exercise has been shown to increase cell sensitivity to insulin, reduce glucose production by the liver and increase utilization of glucose by muscle. Thus there is evidence to suggest that regular exercise can prevent non-insulin-dependent diabetes mellitus (NIDDM) developing in those who have impaired glucose tolerance. Obesity and NIDDM are increasing healthcare problems throughout the Western world and the role for exercise cannot be overstated.

Body composition and weight

Body weight and percentage body fat increase with advancing age. An increase in truncal body fat is closely associated with increased morbidity and earlier mortality. Research has shown that regular exercisers accumulate less fat in central and upper body regions than their sedentary counterparts, with a period of aerobic exercise training leading to loss of body fat predominantly from these areas. It is widely accepted that body weight decreases in those who start to exercise, providing calorie intake does not rise to meet the new demands. Exercise is therefore a vital component of a weight loss programme and healthy living.

Bone responses

The prevalence of osteoporosis increases with advancing age, it being one of the most common conditions affecting postmenopausal women. Morbidity is primarily related to the associated fractures of the neck of femur, vertebrae and wrist. In recent years research has focused on whether certain forms of exercise enhance bone mineral density. Studies are conflicting regarding the benefits of strength training, thought to be the exercise of choice because of the positive relationship between muscle strength and bone mineral density (BMD), which is related to proximal muscle group strength. A recent review concluded that strength training can at least prevent some of the losses in BMD that occur with age. However, the magnitude of these changes is not large enough to prevent a fracture once a fall has occurred. It is more likely that the role of strength training lies in the primary prevention of falls rather than secondary prevention of fracture.

Muscle responses

Muscle mass decreases with age (sarcopenia), with significant consequences. These include an increase in the number of falls and therefore fractures, poor thermoregulation, a reduction in the metabolic rate and loss of functional capacity, thereby decreasing ability to carry out activities of daily living. However, participation of an elderly group in a 2-month strength-training programme reversed at least two decades' decline in strength and muscle mass. This initial change was considered to be mainly due to neural adaptations, leading to increased motor unit firing frequency and maximal motor unit recruitment rates with improved efficiency. With more prolonged resistance training, modest muscle fibre hypertrophy occurs, producing a complete reversal of muscle fibre atrophy in some individuals.

Psychological benefits

The mental health benefits of exercise have not been researched as intensively as the physical benefits. However, there is some evidence to suggest that the following may occur: preserved cognitive function, a decrease in depressive symptoms, improved self-confidence and sense of personal control/independence (Fig. 14.1).

Immune system

An increase in IgG levels in men and a fall in IgM levels in women was demonstrated after a 2-month exercise training programme. Changes were said to be within the normal range and the conclusion was that exercise had beneficial effects. Natural killer cell activity has also been shown to change after exercise:

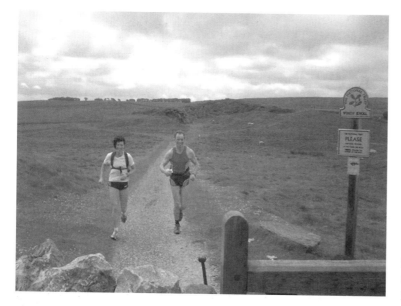

Fig. 14.1 Exercise may preserve cognitive function and improve psychological wellbeing.

the number and activity of these cells in the peripheral blood increased after males with a mean age of 68.5 years regularly practised a particular form of t'ai chi. Further studies are required.

Pre-existing medical conditions

For the vast majority of people over the age of 65, physical activity will be beneficial, although there are conditions where exercise is contraindicated, such as very recent myocardial infarction, unstable angina, severe valvular disease, severe heart failure and uncontrolled metabolic conditions.

As previously discussed the risks and complications of conditions such as type 2 diabetes, cardiovascular disease and osteoporosis, all decrease in association with exercise.

However, with increasing age comes the greater likelihood that these medical conditions will exist and require treatment in the form of medication. It is beyond the scope of this chapter to discuss all relevant medications; however, a few important classes are presented:

• ACE inhibitors work well in the athlete with hypertension as they do not limit V_{O_2}max, whereas beta-blockers, also used in hypertension or additionally for angina and post-myocardial infarction, restrict exercise capacity because they limit increases in heart rate response to exercise and therefore lower

cardiac output. Serum potassium can also increase during exercise in those on beta-blockers, and so should be monitored. One should also be aware of the increased risk of hyperthermia due to impaired blood flow to the skin and vasoconstriction, therefore contraindicating nonselective beta-blockers.

• Diuretics may increase the risks of dehydration and therefore the symptoms of postural hypotension and fainting. They have also been reported to cause cardiac arrhythmias during physical activity, possibly due to hypokalaemia and worsened during bouts of exercise when there are increased levels of catecholamines.

• Calcium channel blockers are also used to treat angina and hypertension, and may impair cardiac output during exercise and therefore lower performance. Nitrates have a similar negative effect, although they can also improve exercise tolerance in some by increasing cardiac blood flow.

• Anxiolytics as a group can affect fine motor skills, coordination, reaction time and thermoregulation, leading to an increased risk of injury.

The American College of Sports Medicine (ACSM) stated in 1998 that a regular exercise programme was an effective way to reduce a number of functional declines associated with ageing. This statement, along with increasing amounts of research showing the benefits of regular exercise in the elderly, has produced a shift in attitudes. Exercise prescription is integral and should be treated like any other therapy, with the benefits, costs and potential side effects being fully evaluated.

Risks of exercise

Exercise has many benefits, but the risks should be considered. These can be broadly categorized into the risk of sudden death and the risk of injury.

Risk of sudden death

Although rare, it is obviously an emotive subject, with the underlying causes differing between younger and older athletes. Over the age of 35 coronary artery disease is the most common cause of sudden death during exercise with incidence rising with age. Population studies recount figures of around 1 death per 15–18 000 exercisers per year (see Chapter 11).

When advising older groups, this risk should be considered but should not put individuals off exercising, as the overall benefits outweigh the risk. The use of pre-participation examination may pick up those most at risk, enabling exercise programmes to be personalized for these individuals. Studies of post-mortem findings following sudden death found that the majority of those who died demonstrated modifiable risk factors for coronary heart disease (CHD) such as high cholesterol.

During the pre-participation examination a thorough history, including smoking status, family history of cardiovascular disease and alcohol intake (the risk factors for CHD), is necessary. A full cardiorespiratory examination and resting electrocardiogram (ECG) are easy to undertake during the screening. Fasting glucose and lipid measurements are also relevant in excluding an increased risk of diabetes or hyperlipidaemia. The ACSM has recommended that treadmill stress tests should be performed on males >40 and females >50 years wishing to take part in vigorous activity (>60% maximal oxygen uptake). Studies have shown that in asymptomatic individuals exercise tolerance tests (ETT) are less sensitive and specific and it is known that most of those who die suddenly have had negative ETTs, whilst many of those with positive ETTs do not have significant disease (i.e. >50% stenosis on angiogram). Echocar-diography is recommended for those who have positive examination findings or symptoms that could be attributed to a cardiac problem. Chapter 11 discusses these difficulties in detail.

Injuries

Vulnerability to injury increases with age as a result of the physiological changes, previously described, that occur within the soft tissues (tendons, ligaments and joint capsules). This increased susceptibility is further compounded by the age-related changes that occur in the process of tissue repair, principally:
- the inflammatory phase is significantly reduced;
- during the proliferative phase cellular migration, proliferation and maturation are delayed;
- during the remodelling phase, collagen is laid down both more sparingly and slowly, with altered binding patterns.

The net result is a delayed and less adequate healing process post-injury.

Osteoarthritis

Osteoarthritis (OA) is present in almost 85% of those aged 85 and over. Characterized by joint pain, stiffness and limitation of movement, the general consensus is that it is a multifactorial illness associated with ageing rather than a necessary consequence of ageing. Other risk factors for osteoarthritis include obesity, gender, trauma, congenital anomalies, genetics and biomechanical factors. The relationship between arthritis and exercise is unclear, but prolonged impact loading is almost certainly a significant risk factor. The general consensus is that sports subjecting joints to high levels of impact and torsional loading increase the risk of articular cartilage degeneration. In contrast, moderate regular exercise does not increase the risk of OA, although studies involving runners have produced conflicting results. In general runners do not develop OA at the hip or knee any more frequently than non-runners, in the absence of previous joint injury. Many studies have demonstrated the benefits of exercise in treating patients with mild to moderate OA, preventing joint stiffness and pain, whilst maintaining muscle strength and proprioception.

Summary

It is obvious that the veteran athlete is different in many ways, on one hand demonstrating a poorer healing rate following injury, whilst on the other benefiting from decreased cardiovascular and musculoskeletal morbidity. Perhaps more importantly, active elderly people are more independent and less reliant upon health and social services. In summary it seems to point towards the view that exercise for all remains the best buy in public health.

Further reading

American College of Sports Medicine Position Stand. Exercise and physical activity for older adults. *Med Sci Sports Exerc* 1998, **30**, 992–1008.

Buckwalter JA, Lane NE. Athletics and osteoarthritis. *Am J Sports Med* 1997, **25**, 873–881.

Karlsson M. Does exercise reduce the burden of fractures? A review. *Acta Orthop Scand* 2002, **73**, 691–705.

Kligman EW, Hewitt MJ, Crowell DL. Recommending exercise to healthy older adults. *The Physician and Sportsmedicine* 1999, **27**, 42–62.

Levine GN, Balady GJ. The benefits and risks of exercise training: The exercise prescription. *Adv Int Med* 1993, **38**, 57–74.

Li JX, Hong Y, Chan KM *et al.* Tai chi: physiological characteristics and beneficial effects on health. *Br J Sports Med* 2001, **35**, 148–156.

Mazzeo RS, Tanaka H. Exercise prescription for the elderly. Current recommendations. *Sports Med* 2001, **31**, 809–818.

Sutton AJ, Muir KR, Mockett S, Fentem P. A case control study to investigate the relation between low and moderate levels of physical activity and osteoarthritis of the knee using data collected as part of the Allied Dunbar National Fitness Survey. *Ann Rheum Dis* 2001, **60**, 756–764.

15 Disability sport

Introduction

Sport for people with disabilities has been an evolving phenomenon for the last half century. From the first 'games' at Stoke Mandeville Hospital in 1948, involving 16 people with spinal cord injury, the Paralympics has progressed to a multidisability event with more than 4000 athletes from about 130 countries, making it one of the largest sporting events in the world. Outstanding performances demonstrate the potential for people with disabilities to excel in their own right, with wheelchair marathon times commonly below one-and-a-half hours! Single leg amputees can clear more than 2 m in the high jump, and recently competed against able-bodied competitors in the 2002 Commonwealth Games swimming events.

Physical activity for health

The development of competitive sport for people with disabilities has raised the awareness of the potential for physical activity for a person with a disability (Box 15.1). This is helping to change attitudes in the medical profession towards physical activity in people with disabilities. The beneficial effects of

---

Box 15.1 Key points

- Large increase in participation in sport/exercise for people with disabilities over last half century.
- Increased awareness of physical capabilities of people despite disability.
- Benefits from physical activity resulting in reduced healthcare costs.
- Important for medical profession to encourage physical activity for health gain.

---

exercise are well established in relation to maintenance of health. In many diseases – e.g. coronary heart disease (CHD), non-insulin-dependent diabetes mellitus (NIDDM) and osteoporosis – physical activity is an integral part of prevention and management of the condition. People with disabilities should be encouraged to remain physically active, but participation in sport is not essential.

The message suggesting at least 30 minutes of moderate intensity activity on at least five days of the week, is equally applicable to someone with a disability. The same principles of training apply, namely the graded increase in duration, intensity and frequency of activity, but more thought may be required as to the mode of exercise according to the disability.

Unfortunately people with disabilities are often not encouraged to seek these benefits for a variety of reasons, including cultural and social factors, as well as access and availability of suitable facilities. The social and psychological benefits derived from exercise and participation in sport are not exclusive to the able-bodied, and significant improvements in self-esteem and social integration are gained through an active lifestyle. Current evidence shows that active people with certain disabilities visit their doctor less frequently, whilst paraplegic athletes are less likely to suffer major medical complications than their nonathletic counterparts.

Organization of sport for people with disabilities

Disabilities present in many forms and may be physical, sensory or intellectual. Consequently there are a number of organizations that promote and support sport for people with disabilities worldwide. The

International Paralympic Committee (IPC), with the exception of the hearing impaired, unites these organizations globally. The hearing impaired hold a games termed the 'deaflympics' every four years staged in a non-Olympic Games year. The Paralympic Games involves sport at the elite level and is held just after, and in the same city as, the Olympic Games for the following disability groups:
- spinal cord-related disability;
- amputees;
- visually impaired (VI);
- cerebral palsy (CP);
- Les Autres – other physical disabilities not falling into the above four categories, e.g. muscular dystrophy, multiple sclerosis;
- intellectual disability (or learning disability).

Sports of the Athens 2004 Paralympic Games were as follows: archery, athletics, boccia (a form of bowling for those with cerebral palsy), cycling, equestrian, football five-a-side, football seven-a-side, goalball (for visually impaired athletes), judo, powerlifting, sailing, shooting, swimming, table tennis, volleyball, wheelchair basketball, wheelchair fencing, wheelchair rugby and wheelchair tennis.

There are also Winter Paralympic Games with Alpine and Nordic events, as well as sledge hockey – a form of ice hockey using a seated sledge.

The Special Olympics is a separate event involving those with an intellectual disability, with less emphasis on elite performance and more on participation.

Advice on choosing a sport/exercise

From the health aspect there are significant differences between exercise for health and sport. Sport is not always exercise and vice versa. Sport implies competition and the physiological demands are determined by the sport; for example, wheelchair sprint racing (anaerobic) vs wheelchair road racing (aerobic) vs pistol shooting (skill). Sport may also involve trauma, which will be particularly undesirable in some medical conditions, for instance osteogenesis imperfecta. Alternatively the focus may be on socialization and building self-esteem. Several factors will need to be considered if advising on a suitable sport:
- Personal preference – important for adherence.
- Characteristics of the sport:
  - physiological demands;
  - collision potential;
  - team or individual;
  - coordination requirements.
- Medical condition – beneficial and detrimental aspects.
- Associated conditions.
- Cognitive ability.
- Social skills of the person – ability to follow rules and interact with others.
- Availability of facilities.
- Availability of appropriate coaching and support staff (e.g. lifting and handling).
- Equipment availability and cost.

At the elite level, wheelchairs are designed particularly for the sport and are not for daily use. Wheelchair racing has derived much of its technology from cycling. Specialist chairs are available for sports such as tennis, rugby and basketball (Fig. 15.1).

The health benefits of exercise are not necessarily achieved through sport, with different sports impos-

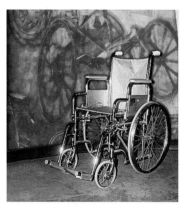
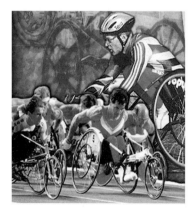

Fig. 15.1 Demonstrates wheelchair designs, specifically for sport.

ing different physiological stresses and injury risks. This aside, many people do derive increases both in fitness and well-being through their sport.

Sports can be classified based upon their aerobic intensity, potential for trauma and coordination demands. An understanding of this classification process helps one appreciate the associated risks and benefits. These factors then have to be married with the individual's medical condition and other considerations such as local facilities.

Each of the different disability groups present different medical problems. Not all disability groups partake in all the sports listed in Table 15.1. For example, judo and goalball are only for the visually impaired, while boccia is only for those with cerebral palsy.

Classification

To try and ensure fair competition, a system of classification exists to place athletes of similar ability against each other. In some sports this will be disability specific; for example in athletics, athletes with the same sort of disability compete against each other. In other sports, for instance swimming, there is a functional classification that places swimmers with different conditions in the same group based upon a static musculoskeletal and neurological assessment, and a dynamic evaluation of participation in the sport. Hence one could see swimmers with

spinal cord injury (SCI), CP and limb deficiencies all in the same race. In team sports, such as wheelchair basketball or rugby, different abilities are scored on a points system and only a certain number of points are allowed on the court at any one time. This ensures that those with higher levels of disability are not excluded from team sports. For further information see www.paralympic.org.

It is important that any classification recognizes the athlete's potential physical capabilities and does not penalize those who perform better through training or skill acquisition. For athletes with an intellectual disability, setting the level at which someone becomes eligible to participate can pose difficulties. Significant impairment in intellectual functioning is generally classed as an IQ score of 75 or lower, with significant limitations in, for example, communication and social/interpersonal skills and these must be evident before 18 years of age. This makes it impossible for the athlete to compete 'on reasonably equal terms' with nondisabled athletes. As such this is open to subjective interpretation and has been abused in the past. The Spanish basketball team in the Sydney Paralympic games were later found to have no disability and their gold medals were removed.

The disability groups

Disability groups are as follows:

Table 15.1 Examples of sports collision potential, aerobic intensity and coordination needs

Collision or contact potential	Limited contact potential	Non-contact
Judo	Athletics	Archery
Basketball	Volleyball	Table tennis
Alpine skiing	Nordic skiing	Shooting
High aerobic intensity	Moderate aerobic intensity	Low aerobic intensity
Athletics	Equestrian	Archery
Nordic skiing	Table tennis	Boccia
Swimming	Judo	Bowling
High coordination	Moderate coordination	Low coordination
Basketball	Volleyball	Powerlifting
Shooting	Goalball	Athletics – track
Archery	Soccer	Boccia

Adapted from American Academy of Pediatrics 1982.

- spinal cord-related disability;
- amputees;
- visually impaired;
- cerebral palsy;
- Les Autres;
- intellectual disability.

Spinal cord-related disability

This may be congenital (e.g. spina bifida) or acquired (e.g. trauma or disease). Of the spinally injured, 60% are in the 16–30 age group with a male to female ratio of 4:1. The majority of these are related to road traffic accidents (RTAs), with about 15% occurring in sport, particularly diving, rugby, horse riding and skiing. The injuries are classified by considering the level of neurological loss and whether the lesion is complete or partial (incomplete paralysis) (Fig. 15.2).

Spinal injury results in a number of problems:
- Motor loss – loss of muscle function relating to the level of injury.
- Sensory loss – increasing the risk of pressure sores.

- Loss of autonomic control, e.g. sweating, affecting thermoregulation.
- Respiratory function – loss of intercostal muscle function.
- Effects on cardiac function in exercise (Fig. 15.3) – sympathectomized myocardium in higher spinal lesions gives reduced maximum heart rate of 110–130 beats/min.
- There is limited:
  - cardioacceleration;
  - myocardial contractility;
  - stroke volume;
  - cardiac output.

Amputee or limb deficiency

This may be congenital (e.g. developmental) or acquired. Acquired lesions are usually due to:
- disease – e.g. tumour, vascular disease;
- trauma – RTA, workplace injury.

An athlete with a limb deficiency may compete:
1 With a prosthesis, e.g. running (Fig. 15.4).
2 Without a prosthesis, e.g. swimming, high jump.
3 In a wheelchair, e.g. tennis, basketball.

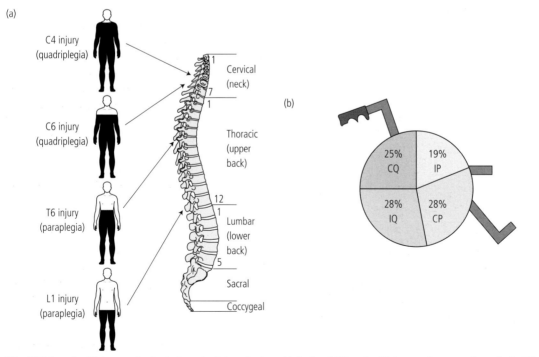

(a)

C4 injury (quadriplegia)

C6 injury (quadriplegia)

T6 injury (paraplegia)

L1 injury (paraplegia)

1
Cervical (neck)
7
1
Thoracic (upper back)
12
1
Lumbar (lower back)
5
Sacral
Coccygeal

(b)

25% CQ | 19% IP
28% IQ | 28% CP

Fig. 15.2 Levels of injury and extent of paralysis in spinal cord injuries. (a) Levels of injury and extent of paralysis. (b) Values by % complete/incomplete paraplegia/quadriplegia.

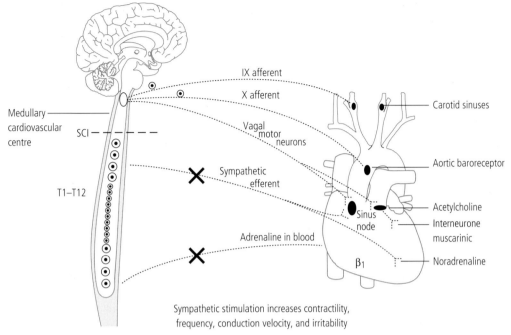

Fig. 15.3 Control of cardiac function.

Sport-specific prostheses enable improved athletic performance with enhanced return of energy after foot strike to mimic the function of the normal Achilles tendon. The fitting and alignment of the prosthesis is important for both function and reducing the risk of musculoskeletal injury. Impact injury or skin chafing of the residual limb are common problems.

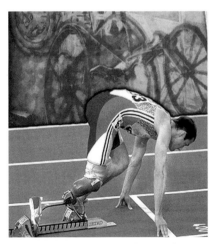

Fig. 15.4 Athlete may compete with a prosthesis, e.g. in running.

Cerebral palsy

Cerebral palsy is a group of disorders affecting body movement and muscle coordination and is caused by an insult or anomaly of the developing brain. Any impairment of brain development, whether of genetic or developmental origin, or the result of injury or disease, may result in cerebral palsy. Cerebral palsy may be classified according to the number of limbs affected and/or by the type of movement disorder (Fig. 15.5).

• Spastic cerebral palsy – is the most common type and is caused by damage to the motor cortex. Spastic muscles are tight and stiff, limiting movement.

• Choreo-athetoid cerebral palsy – results from damage to the basal ganglia or cerebellum and leads to difficulty in controlling and coordinating movement.

• Mixed-type cerebral palsy – occurs when areas of the brain influencing both muscle tone and voluntary movement are affected.

The classification of the movement disorder and number of limbs involved are usually combined (e.g. 'spastic diplegia').

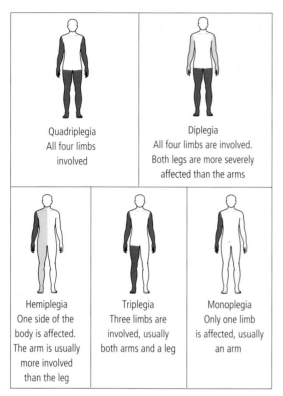

Quadriplegia
All four limbs
involved

Diplegia
All four limbs are involved.
Both legs are more severely
affected than the arms

Hemiplegia
One side of the
body is affected.
The arm is usually
more involved
than the leg

Triplegia
Three limbs are
involved, usually
both arms and a leg

Monoplegia
Only one limb
is affected, usually
an arm

Fig. 15.5 Classification of cerebral palsy by affected limbs.

Athletes with CP commonly have associated problems, namely:
• epilepsy;
• visual defects;
• deafness;
• intellectual impairment.

Approximately half of athletes with CP compete in wheelchairs. The spasticity associated with the condition may be important for function, and without that tone the athlete might not be able to, for example, stabilize his or her trunk. Hence the normal practice of stretching pre-exercise may not be appropriate for all athletes with CP. Maintaining range of movement with flexibility exercises is important, but may have to be done away from the competitive environment.

Visually impaired

Visually impaired athletes are classified using ophthalmological examination, reflecting both visual acuity and field of vision:

Class B1 – a total absence of perception of light in both eyes, or some perception of light but with an inability to recognize the form of a hand at any distance and in any direction.

Class B2 – ranges from the ability to recognize the form of a hand to a visual acuity of 2/60 and/or a visual field of less than 5°.

Class B3 – ranges from a visual acuity of above 2/60 to a visual acuity of 6/60 and/or a visual field or more than 5° and less than 20°.

All classifications must be made by measuring the best eye and to the highest possible correction. This means that all athletes who normally use contact lenses or correcting glasses must wear them during classification, whether or not they intend to use them during competition.

Sports for the visually impaired include athletics, judo and swimming. In cycling a sighted pilot rider is used on a tandem. Guide runners or callers may be used in athletics. In biathlon the skier will follow a guide skier and use a rifle that produces a high tone when aimed at the centre of the target for the shooting component of the event. Injuries in visually impaired athletes often occur following falls, collisions or misplaced footing.

Les Autres

This group encompasses a variety of physical disabilities that do not fit easily within a specific category and includes a number of conditions, such as:
• congenital disorders – e.g. spondylo-epiphyseal dysplasia, Stickler syndrome;
• limb deficiencies;
• muscular dystrophies;
• multiple sclerosis;
• ankylosis or arthritis of major joints.

The variety of conditions and in particular the variety of rare syndromes encountered in disability sport, makes the care of these athletes a challenge for the physician.

Intellectual disability

In the main these athletes are able-bodied, unless the disability results from a head injury, for example, when there may be associated physical changes. As such they are susceptible to the same sport-related injuries as able-bodied athletes. However, the challenge for the treating doctor is in taking the history and then explaining the diagnosis and management of the condition and supervising the rehabilitation. Training errors are more common and correcting technical problems may be more difficult. Athletes with an intellectual disability may be over keen to please their coach in training and may be susceptible to abusive practices. The 'duty of care issues' are important with these athletes.

Elite sport profiling

In able-bodied sport there is a large body of evidence based on the profiles of the physical characteristics of elite athletes to help in the identification of future champions. Although elite disability sport is gaining more credibility worldwide, there is still a shortage of research and documentation relating to these athletes' performance capabilities, making talent identification and profiling more difficult. This is compounded by:

• multiple disability groups that may take part within a single sport;
• wide range of abilities within the same disability, e.g. different levels of spinal injury;
• different physiological responses to exercise, e.g. paraplegics vs quadriplegics;
• concurrent illness, which may interfere with a regular training capability;
• research is related more to rehabilitation and/or exercise therapy than performance related;
• limited exposure to good-quality coaching.

Aspects of 'wheelchair physiology'

Comparisons of the physiology in wheelchair athletes to non-disabled cyclists are made with cycling rather than running, because of the ability to roll and coast without pushing at times. The push frequency relates to the push economy and is individual to the athlete. Propulsion techniques vary between athletes and therefore there is much more variation in performance. Physiological testing may be performed on a modified treadmill or field testing may use a modified 'bleep' (multistage fitness) test to assess aerobic capacity (Fig. 15.6).

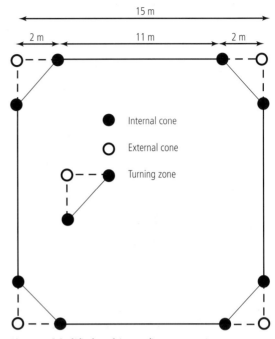

Fig. 15.6 Modified multistage fitness test course.

Injury

Injuries may be sport specific or disability specific (Box 15.2). Some injuries are more common in certain disability groups, for example hand injuries in wheelchair athletes. Alternatively the disability may cause other factors that predispose towards injury.

Disuse osteoporosis in the legs of the paraplegic, for example, will mean that minimal trauma may result in fracture. A fall from the chair in, say, wheelchair basketball can result in a fracture, although the trauma might appear to be low impact. Signs of swelling and deformity may be the only clue if sensation is absent. It could result in autonomic dysreflexia (see later) and this might be the only sign.

Box 15.2 Injuries

• Sport-specific injuries.
• Disability-specific injuries.
• Disuse osteoporosis.
• Remember to think about conditions associated with syndromes.

It is important to consider all the implications that certain syndromes may have on injury risk. An athlete may be competing because of, say, a visual impairment 'Stickler syndrome'; however, the syndrome may also have implications as regards collagen healing and tissue repair.

It is beyond the scope of this chapter to discuss these injuries in detail, but one should definitely think of the increased challenges posed in managing the rehabilitation following, for instance, anterior cruciate ligament (ACL) rupture of a visually impaired athlete.

Not surprisingly upper limb injuries predominate in the wheelchair athlete. The most common ones include:

- soft tissue injuries;
- blisters;
- skin lacerations and abrasions;
- symptoms of hand weakness or numbness.

The repetitive and forceful hand movements and pressure with the heel of the hand on the push rim of the chair may result in peripheral nerve entrapments. The median nerve at the carpal tunnel is most frequently affected, followed by the ulnar nerve at the wrist and forearm.

A high incidence of shoulder pain has been reported in wheelchair athletes; however, these findings have largely been a result of self-reporting and/or questionnaires. Shoulder symptoms were the most common presentation in the Great Britain squad before and during the Atlanta Paralympic Games in 1996; however, on clinical assessment, cervicothoracic dysfunction was the finding most responsible for these symptoms. Clearly shoulder pain does not necessarily mean shoulder pathology and caution should be applied when reviewing the results of 'self-report' studies. Wheelchair athletes involved with overhead activities such as tennis, swimming, basketball and field throwing sports, are more likely to present with true shoulder pathology, such as rotator cuff pathology and impingement syndromes. The mechanics involved in wheelchair propulsion do not in themselves involve sufficient levels of shoulder abduction commonly to give rise to the above mentioned symptoms. However, various other factors predispose the paralympic athlete to spinal pain and shoulder pathology, including:

- existing spinal disease/injury;
- scoliosis +/- spasm;
- sport-specific factors;
- visual impairment – tend to adopt protracted chin posture;
- seating posture in wheelchair;
- protracted shoulders from push position;
- muscle imbalance.

Thermoregulation

The spinally injured athlete has impaired thermoregulation, which may impair performance or increase the risk of heat-related illness. There are several factors contributing to this:

- loss of peripheral receptor function;
- loss of autonomic control on the sweating effector mechanism;
- loss of control of vasoconstriction or vasodilatation of the peripheral vasculature.

The extent of the problem relates to the level of the spinal cord injury and the lowermost functioning sympathetic nervous components. Spinal reflex sweating below the level of the spinal lesion is minimal and is insufficient to regulate body temperature during thermal stress or exercise. However, during exercise in the heat a quadriplegic's sweat rate above level of lesion can rise sixfold. This sweat drips off and is therefore ineffective in assisting through evaporative heat loss. The basal sweat rate below the lesion is unaffected by activity or ambient temperature.

Similar problems occur in the cold with an inability to detect falling core temperature until critical points are reached. Anticipation and preparation for the environment are important factors for the medical care of the disabled athlete.

Team travel issues

Doctors travelling with a team of athletes with disabilities will need to plan carefully for their trip. A detailed medical history of all athletes will help in assessing the risks and additional equipment or medications required. For example, there is a higher prevalence of epilepsy in athletes with a disability. The additional equipment required (sports chair, throwing frame for field events, etc.) places an additional burden on the accompanying staff, with lifting and handling implications. The accessibility, or lack of, to toilets on aircraft discourages intake of adequate fluids to maintain hydration, and athletes may arrive in a dehydrated state after long flights. Dehydration may lead to the exacerbation of urinary tract infection or urinary calculi in the spinally injured athlete. Long-haul flights and coach journeys increase the risk of pressure sores in those without sensation. The risk of deep vein thrombosis is now a known risk with air travel and the disabled athlete may be unable to move around and stretch on the plane. Dependent oedema may also occur after long flights.

Autonomic dysreflexia

This condition occurs in people with spinal cord lesions of T6 level and above. It is triggered by nociceptive (painful) input below the level of the lesion, such as an ingrowing toenail, urinary calculi or anal fissure. Sensory impulses enter the cord below the lesion and the sympathetic nervous system responds to local spinal reflexes with an excessive discharge that is uncorrected. There are inappropriate amounts of noradrenaline (norepinephrine) released, producing hypertension, sweating and headache. It may result in severe hypertension and there are recorded cases of cerebral haemorrhage, fits and deaths reported from hospital patients. Fortunately there are no reported serious consequences from use in athletes.

'Boosting' is a term used to reflect the intentional induction of a dysreflexic state to enhance athletic performance. Athletes with a spinal injury found that it felt easier to push harder when in the dysreflexic state, and started to use techniques to bring this about, for example clamping a catheter to produce bladder distension, tight leg straps, or prolonged sitting in the racing chair. Research showed that treadmill exercise capability improved, as did simulated race times by nearly 10% when in the 'boosted' state. Concerns were raised that these athletes were putting themselves at risk. No adverse events have been seen in an athletic situation and it is possible that the increased cardiovascular fitness in the athletic population has a protective effect. Initially the practice was deemed a doping offence, but it is now

considered a health issue and athletes suspected of boosting may have their blood pressure checked pre-race, which if elevated above 160 mmHg systolic or 90 mmHg diastolic can result in withdrawal from the event.

Doping issues

The International Paralympic Committee have signed up to the World Anti-Doping Code list of substances and prohibited methods in 2004. Doping offences have been seen in disability sport and although it is clear some cases have been intentional, it is well recognized that a far greater proportion of athletes with disabilities will be taking prescribed medication and that the family physician may have a poor knowledge of doping regulations. Chronic pain, hypertension and renal disease are common conditions requiring treatment in disabled athletes. Allowances are made in the collection procedure, allowing supervision for visually impaired or intellectually impaired athletes. Athletes requiring catheters, using condom drainage or having severe disabilities may use a larger collection vessel and use their own catheters.

Summary

The performances achieved by athletes with disabilities continue to amaze. Additionally the sports medicine challenges they create for the doctor require an understanding of the sport and the disability-specific issues, and the ability flexibly to apply sports medicine practices established through able-bodied experiences.

Further reading

Fallon KE. The disabled athlete. In: Bloomfield J, Fricker PA, Fitch KD (eds) *Science and Medicine in Sport*. Carlton, Blackwell Science, 1995, pp. 550–551.

Webborn ADJ. Sports in children with physical disabilities/ Medical problems of disabled child athletes. In: Maffulli N, Chan KM, Macdonald R, Malina RM, Parker AW (eds) *Sports Medicine for Specific Ages and Abilities*. Edinburgh, Churchill Livingstone, 2001.

16 Sports-specific injuries

Soccer

Soccer is the world's most popular team game, with a reported 200 million participants. Because of its physical nature, it has been described as a 'collision sport'. However, the sport involves different demands, which are position dependent and so vary between goalkeeper, full-back, central defender, midfield and attack.

A typical player will be involved in the following activities during a match:
- jogging 40%
- walking 25%
- cruising 15%
- sprinting 10%
- backwards movement 10%

A player may only be in possession of the ball for as little as 2 minutes.

Injury epidemiology

Injuries most commonly occur during a tackle (23.5%), with twice as many injuries being sustained by the player being tackled (15.4%), compared with the tackler (8.1%). The majority of other injuries are related to running (20.0%), twisting/turning (8.1%) and shooting (5.9%). Soccer training sessions involve significantly less tackling and contact than matches, and this is reflected in the majority of collision injuries occurring during matches. Non-collision injuries appear to be evenly distributed between training and matches.

Training injuries occur more commonly during the traditional pre-season conditioning phase of a season. These injuries, which are predominantly of an overuse nature involving soft tissues, were reduced in one premier league club from 21 in one season

to 2 during the following three years by decreasing the running load on the players and involving other non-running strategies for improving fitness. A subsequent running-based aerobic fitness test (intermittent Yo-Yo test) demonstrated no deterioration in fitness following a change in training.

The trend is for training injuries to gradually decrease throughout the season, with match injuries, which have a high occurrence during the first four months of the season, also declining by approximately 50% in the second half of the season.

Site of injury

Over 80% of all soccer injuries involve soft tissues (muscle, ligament, tendon). The most common sites are listed in Table 16.1. The majority of muscular injuries in the thigh affect the hamstrings, with approximately 50% fewer injuries being sustained to the quadriceps and adductor muscle groups.

Table 16.1 The most common sites involved in soccer injuries

Location	Percent
Thigh	23.4
Ankle	18.5
Knee	15.1
Groin	9.8
Calf	8.2
Foot	4.9
Lumbar spine	4.4
Lower leg	3.1
Hip	2.6
Other	10.1

The anterior talofibular ligament of the ankle is the most commonly injured ligamentous structure, with a frequency of more than twice that of injury to the medial collateral ligament of the knee.

Predisposing factors for injury

In addition to the usual intrinsic predisposing risks for injury, such as previous injury history, age, biomechanics, height and weight, there are additional soccer-specific positional factors (Table 16.2). Injuries appear to be more common during matches as each half progresses, with more injuries occurring in each successive 15-minute period. This pattern is also present in training, and fatigue would therefore appear to be a major contributing factor in soccer injuries.

The equipment used in soccer that may have an impact on injuries needs to be considered, in particular shin guards and boots, of which there are various designs. Players will often not wear shin guards in training, and also use different boots than those chosen on match day. Further studies need to be undertaken into the effects of equipment on injuries in soccer.

Effect of injury

An 'audit of injuries in professional football' was performed during the seasons 1997–1999 and demonstrated that an average injury in the English Premier League resulted in a player missing 23.95 training days and 3.43 matches. This translates to a substantial cost to the professional game. Various injury prevention strategies have been tried, and in one premier league club over a three-year period, the average loss per injury was reduced to 16.3 training days and 2.39 matches by introducing simple changes to the training regime.

Table 16.2 Playing positions in soccer and their associated injury rate

Playing position	Percent injuries
Goalkeeper	6.9
Defence	40.5
Midfield	29.2
Attack	23.4

Injuries requiring operative management

Of the more commonly occurring procedures, arthroscopic intervention undertaken for meniscal or chondral damage appears to figure prominently. Although soft tissue injuries are the most frequent occurrence in soccer, meniscal injuries cause great concern, as a result of the studies demonstrating the future development of osteoarthritis in the knee. Many former professional soccer players report painful knees affecting their activities of daily living. Where technically possible, a policy of performing meniscal repair rather than resection, in order to try to preserve meniscus and prevent the development of osteoarthritis, should be followed (see Chapter 7). Although short-term recovery in terms of return to competition is significantly longer following meniscal repair, one should question the ethics of meniscal resection purely on the basis of a rapid return to competition.

Explorations of the Achilles tendon are often undertaken alongside stripping of the paratenon, and are a reasonably frequent occurrence due to the presence of Achilles tendinosis (see Chapter 8). The number of chronic Achilles injuries is a reflection of the nature of soccer, which involves a combination of running and plyometric activity. Sportsman's hernia is a common problem in soccer. It is hypothesized that the twisting/turning nature of the sport, combined with the use of the adductors as hip flexors when kicking the ball, puts a shearing force across the abdomen causing a vulnerability to osteitis pubis in the developing skeleton or groin disruption where there is greater skeletal maturity (see Chapter 6).

Soccer is the 'beautiful game', enjoyed by many people throughout the world, and it has been said more than once that 'it's not a matter of life or death; it's more important than that'. Whilst the financial rewards can be great in the elite professional game, there is considerable risk of injury, which may have long-term effects. Simple injury prevention strategies are important for all soccer players of all ages and ability.

Further reading

Ekstrand J, Gillquist J. The avoidability of soccer injuries. *Int J Sports Med* 1983, **4**, 124–128.

Ekstrand J, Gillquist J. Soccer injuries and their mechanism: a prospective study. *Med Sci Sports Exerc* 1983, **15**, 267–270.

Fevre DJ. *Collision Sports: Injury and Repair.* Oxford, Butterworth Heinemann, 1998.

Gibbon WW. Groin pain in professional soccer: A comparison of England and the rest of Western Europe. *Br J Sports Med* 1999, **33**, 435.

Hawkins RD, Hulse MA, Wilkinson C *et al.* The association medical research programme: an audit of injuries in professional football. *Br J Sports Med* 2001, **35**, 43–47.

Track and field

Track and field is an unusual arena to work in because of the diversity of its participants. In the consultation room one may be addressing the medical issues of an underweight, osteoporotic marathon runner presenting with a stress fracture, whilst the next athlete in the waiting room is a 20-stone shot-putter with extension impingement pain of the throwing elbow. This creates a fascinating work environment, but one has to appreciate that this is not so much a team but a collection of individuals each with their own focus. Injury and illness, although commonplace, are a total inconvenience to the athlete, who will not receive funding/money unless he or she is fit and performing on a weekly basis. These athletes will push themselves to physical and psychological limits in order to achieve the ultimate goal, for some an Olympic gold medal or world record (Fig. 16.1). They are therefore a very motivated breed with a tendency to overtrain and ignore 'niggly' injuries unless the coach and/or medical team can directly intervene.

Certain track and field events appear to carry an increased injury risk. In the UK the 400 m runners, the flat jumpers and the endurance athletes generally demand a higher level of medical intervention. Lower limb injuries are commonly present, even in events such as the throws, where one may assume that the upper limb is more at risk.

The four most common medical problems within the sport are:
- upper respiratory tract infection;
- amenorrhoea;
- iron deficiency with low-grade anaemia;
- anxiety-related disorders in association with illness and lack of performance.

Therefore for the purposes of this chapter the five most common injuries occurring in track and field will be discussed, along with the events that present with these problems:
1 Achilles tendinopathy.
2 Infrapatellar tendinopathy.
3 The hamstring 'strain'.
4 Tibialis posterior dysfunction.
5 Mechanical dysfunction of the lumbar spine.

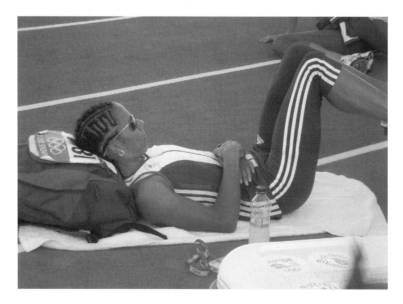

Fig. 16.1 Athletes will push themselves to their physical limits to achieve their ultimate goal.

Achilles tendinopathy

Presentation

Jumpers, javelin throwers, bend runners (200 m up to 1500 m) and endurance runners are affected. The Achilles acts like a coiled spring and it is an effective shock absorber as well as an 'energy return' device to assist with forward and upward propulsion. As with all soft tissue injuries, prevention is better than cure.

The debate continues about what causes the pain with this disorder. Unless there is purely a para-tendinitis, there appears to be little evidence that inflammation is the cause of the pain. But then some respond very well to anti-inflammatory treatment – icing, nonsteroidal anti-inflammatory drugs (NSAIDs) and cortisone injections. Other suggestions are neovascular engorgement, mucinoid degenerative change and oedema within the tendon (see Chapter 8).

Classically this is an overuse injury and its recurrence in the sport can blight an athlete's career. Rehabilitation of this tendon is crucial to prevent recurrence. Power within the gastrocnemius/soleus complex is crucial to 'take the load off' the tendon.

Further details about presentation and management of this condition have already been given in Chapter 8. Surgery certainly has its place in those cases that fail the rehabilitation process. However, in track and field athletes, despite choosing surgeons with great care, the first operation is often found to be the first of several and return to previous performance levels occurs in only 50% of those operated upon.

Of course all the above makes randomized double-blind controlled trials impossible. So, for example, finding a cohort of elite triple jumpers on which to perform evidence-based work would be out of the question. As a doctor in this sport one has to work within the realms of anecdote, possibilities and intuition as well as evidence-based medicine.

Patellar tendinopathy

Presentation

Patellar tendinopathy affects principally flat jumpers, javelin throwers, and endurance and middle distance runners. This so-called 'jumper's knee' is a frustrating complaint for the athlete, as the pain is of a level where the athlete feels that recovery will be rapid and that training is possible (which it may well be but then the question is 'how much?'). The aetiology and pathologies involved are similar to those discussed in relation to the Achilles tendon (see Chapter 7). Studies have shown that this tendon, like the Achilles, evolves as a response to exercise. It is not understood whether this change is purely adaptive and when it becomes detrimental to the performance of the extensor mechanism of the knee. Certainly an asymptomatic pathology in this area seems to be quite normal in jumpers. One tends to address the changes when symptoms develop.

In track and field athletes the history may be one of symptoms brought on during a stage of the season, when the athlete has increased a load on the structure, such as increased weight training, endurance training or plyometrics (an exercise that involves bounding, which is a forceful eccentric manoeuvre producing power whilst the muscle is lengthening; this exercise has been proven to produce high performance levels in those who can tolerate the training). Video analysis can also be used to examine the movements of the tendon and the patella when running and jumping. Further management issues and protocols have been discussed in Chapter 7.

The hamstring strain

Presentation

It is important to determine whether the hamstring has suffered a local tear or whether the 'strain' sensation is a referred pain, from the lumbar spine, for example. The sight of a 100 m sprinter 'pulling up' clutching his or her hamstring is a familiar one. However, on occasions you will see the same athlete competing later on that day or the following day. Clearly they had not sustained a local tear otherwise there would be too much pain and inhibition to perform. This scenario often suggests a neural component to the athlete's pain, that is, pain referred from the spine. A pinch or momentary compression or low-grade irritation of a lower lumbar nerve root may result in muscle hypertonia and a sensation of 'pulling'. As this neural component is not consistent with true neural compromise, imaging is often fruitless, with the disorder being that of a functional problem not a structural one. The athlete may have been suffering for days or weeks with sensations of tightness on that side.

Management

The diagnosis and management of this condition have already been summarized in Chapter 6.

There is no doubt that an accelerated rehabilitation of muscular injuries is allowing return to sport at an earlier stage (see Chapter 18). Once bleeding at the site of injury has subsided then gentle exercise may be considered. Track and field athletes are running again approximately four days following a grade I/II injury to the hamstring.

Other treatments. Hamstring injuries may present in a number of ways, sometimes with recurrent tightness being the only symptomatology. Examination may suggest that the lumbar spine is implicated, with positive neural tension signs and increased hypertonia of the musculature on the affected side. In this situation caudal epidural (injection of corticosteroid and local anaesthetic via the sacral hiatus) is often an adjunct to local treatment.

Local injection therapy is becoming more widely recognized in the field of elite sport, utilizing various homeopathic remedies in an attempt to accelerate healing. Although more research is required in this area, results appear encouraging.

Tibialis posterior dysfunction

Presentation

There is no doubt that dysfunction of this muscle is a disaster for foot, ankle and lower limb function. The condition may present with symptoms directly related to the muscle; however, weakness may not be detected until there is a problem within the foot or lower leg, that may initially appear to be unrelated to the tibialis posterior.

With dysfunction the resulting and progressive planovalgus deformity (and later forefoot abduction) is an avoidable problem if prompt diagnosis of early dysfunction is made. All too often, however, this is not the case because of failure to make an accurate diagnosis.

Tibialis posterior produces plantarflexion and inversion of the ankle and rear foot. It performs this manoeuvre by locking the midtarsal joints and causing a transfer of plantarflexion forces to the metatarsals. Failure to perform this function results in rear foot eversion, the midtarsal area does not lock and therefore the plantarflexion forces act on the talonavicular joint and the medial ligamentous structures thus producing a flat-foot deformity. Tibialis posterior also acts with other muscles to produce a co-contraction of forces about the ankle to add to the stability of the ankle joint.

Symptoms are often noted towards its insertion at the navicular. The tendon also inserts onto the three cuneiforms, the base of the second, third and fourth metatarsals and a further attachment to the inferior calcaneonavicular ligament.

The tendon has an area of hypovascularity proximal to the sustentaculum tali, in addition to there being a bowstring effect due to the tethering action of the flexor retinaculum. The above two factors are further reasons as to why excessive loading produces chronic inflammatory changes in this tendon in a biomechanically inefficient foot and ankle.

The tendon may become symptomatic as a consequence of direct trauma or as a result of an overuse injury. The history is of medial foot pain exacerbated by exercise. There is tenderness and swelling along the path of the tendon. The lower limb biomechanics must be assessed on standing and with the patient walking, as notable overpronation may be the cause of the problem.

Early diagnosis of the condition and its aetiology is the key to success. Active resisted movements may demonstrate weakness, and the tendon may not be palpable in the case of a rupture. Forefoot abduction may be observed by the 'too many toes' sign when visualizing the patient from behind.

Another useful test for this condition is the one foot raise test. The patient stands on the affected leg only and then attempts to heel raise (Fig. 16.2). This will demonstrate a degree of weakness and pain along the medial border of the foot. In severe tibialis posterior tendinosis/rupture, this manoeuvre may not be possible. This would normally be associated with longstanding rear foot abnormalities such as a rear foot valgus, which produces a diseased and elongated tendon. Stages of tibialis posterior tendon degeneration are shown in Table 16.3.

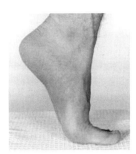

Fig. 16.2 'One foot raise test'.

Investigation

1 Weight-bearing X-rays may demonstrate collapse of the medial foot joints.
2 Ultrasound scan may demonstrate intra- or extra-substance tear of the tendon. The dynamic aspect of this investigation is useful to assess areas of tethering.
3 Magnetic resonance imaging (MRI) scan provides information about the contour of the tendon and is also more precise with regards to the extent of intra-substance pathology. Staging of the disease process correlates well with MRI findings.

Treatment of the condition may therefore entail the use of an orthosis to correct any abnormal biomechanics (particularly to correct the rear foot valgus), local modalities to alleviate the inflammation and a cessation or reduction of the aggravating activities. After a period of relative rest, a rehabilitation regime of lower limb flexibility and a graded return to weight-bearing exercise should be recommended.

In severe disorders immobilization for up to 4 weeks can be considered, with a lower leg brace to create a degree of rear foot inversion and foot plantarflexion.

The presence of chronic intra-substance tendon change prompts consideration of surgery, before the deformity becomes too severe.

Mechanical dysfunction of the lumbar spine

This problem is covered in Chapter 9.

Cricket

Cricketing injuries

Cricket at its best is an ethereal sport to watch, and yet it has been deemed one of the most injury-prone non-contact sports. Fast bowlers are particularly at risk, repeatedly delivering a 5½ ounce missile, at speeds of up to 100 m.p.h., at a batsman wearing body armour and no more than 22 yards away. The bowler absorbs ground reaction forces (GRFs) of up to nine times body weight during delivery stride, the batsman fending off the ball using a bat weighing 2–3 lbs, with a cordon of fielders, both close in and in the deep, all without hand protection bar the wicketkeeper. Fast bowlers are the workhorses of cricket, and among bowlers, batsmen, fielders and wicket-keepers they are the most injury prone (Box 16.1).

Table 16.3 Stages of tibialis posterior tendon degeneration

	Stage 1	Stage 2	Stage 3	Stage 4
Condition of tendon	Tendonitis and/or degeneration	Elongation	Elongation	Rupture
Rearfoot	Mobile. Normal alignment	Mobile valgus position	Fixed valgus position	Fixed valgus position
Pain	Medial, focal and mild	Medial along the tendon and moderate	Medial sometimes lateral and moderate	Medial sometimes lateral and moderate
Heel raise test	Mild weakness	Moderate weakness	Marked weakness	Inability to perform
'Too many toes' sign	Normal	Positive	Positive	Positive
Pathology	Synovial proliferation, degeneration	Moderate degeneration	Marked degeneration	Rupture and marked degeneration

Cricket throws up a delicious blend of traumatic, acute and overuse injuries (Box 16.2), and 'knowing the sport', and 'what they do and how they do it', are the keys to managing them effectively.

Many of the injuries sustained in cricket are no different to any other sport (and are well covered by standard texts), but there are certain injuries that cricketers sustain regularly that are intimately linked to what they do, and how they do it, as detailed below.

Spondylolysis in fast bowlers

Lower back pain in an adolescent fast bowler, of more than 3 months' duration, with clinical signs in extension (positive one-legged extension test, positive Fitch test) is a stress fracture until proven otherwise

Presentation

Lower back pain accounts for 14% of all injuries in cricket and 24% of all missed days. Stress fractures account for 2% of all injuries but 11% of all days lost. Most fast bowlers in any elite bowling squad will have had at least one stress fracture on their way to the top of the game. Some will have had more than one (some get serial fractures), and in certain cases the condition will finish the bowler's career. The adolescent fast bowler is vulnerable, particularly if they bowl with incorrect bowling technique, and are overbowled.

The majority of stress fractures occur at L5 and L4, but L3 is not that uncommon. Beware the bowler

with chronic bilateral pars defects at L5 with fresh acute lesions above at L4 or L3. Lesions may be at the pars, pedicle or lamina. Rarely do they occur above L3, and as a rule, left-armers get right-sided lesions, and right-armers get left-sided lesions. Stress lesions may occur at multiple levels and, like any sport, they may progress to delayed union or nonunion and slip (spondylolisthesis).

It is difficult to sustain a fast-bowling career with a 'listhesis', but not unknown in elite spin bowlers. The symptoms are those of classic bone stress (crescendo pain), with extension-orientated clinical signs (positive one-legged extension test, positive Fitch test; Fig. 16.3). The diagnosis is often not difficult at all, and may be confirmed by single photon emission computed tomography (SPECT) + spiral CT, or by pars MRI + spiral CT (planar bone scanning is relatively insensitive in this context and will miss a significant percentage of early lesions) (Fig. 16.4).

The latter algorithm involves less ionizing radiation – an important factor when imaging adolescent sportsmen or women. The key is to have a high index of suspicion to ensure prompt diagnosis of a potentially reversible lesion that could be healed with appropriate management.

Management

This entails activity modification, rehabilitation involving intensive strengthening with a focus on

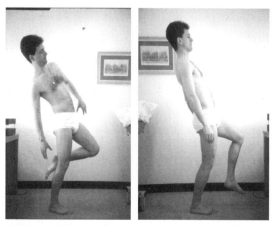

Fig. 16.3 (a) The one-legged extension test is positive when pain is reproduced on the ipsilateral, weight-bearing side on lumbar spine extension. (b) The Fitch test is positive when pain is reproduced on extension positive side rotation towards the ipsilateral, weight bearing side.

(a)

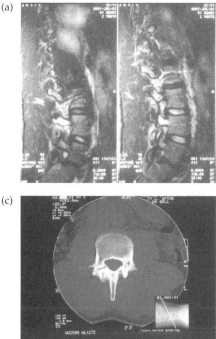

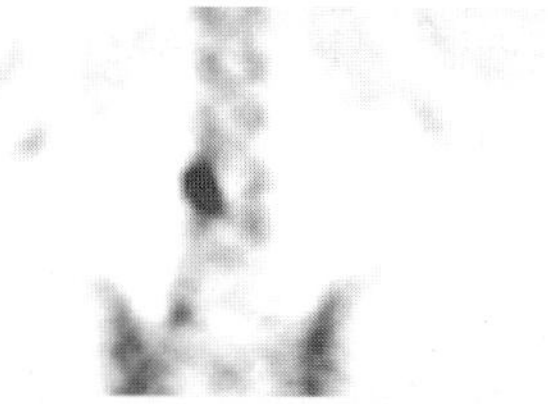

(c)

(b)

Fig 16.4 (a) Pars MRI of the lumbar spine. Intense bone marrow oedema in the left pedicle of L4 in a 17-year-old, right arm, county fast bowler, with bowling-related left-sided low back pain. (b) SPECT scan of the lumbar spine. Multiple lesions at multiple levels. Coronal posterior image of an acute left-sided pedicle stress fracture at L3, and residual low level activity in an old healing lesion of the left L5 pars interarticularis. This right arm, international fast bowler suffered lesions at L5, then L4, and then L3, the latter finishing his career. (c) CT scan of the third lumbar vertebra. Multiple lesions at a single level: a healing stress fracture of the right pars interarticularis and an incomplete stress fracture through the left pedicle, with excellent potential for healing, in an international fast bowler.

core stability, alongside correction of faulty bowling technique and bowling prescription on return to play. The use of bracing to limit extension is controversial. The author's practice is not to brace routinely. Some will come to surgery, most commonly for established lesions bilaterally, with or without spondylolisthesis.

Pivotal to any management strategy is consideration of bowling technique and bowling workload as key aetiological factors: a close working relationship with the coach is therefore vital.

Bowling technique. Certain bowling techniques have been shown to predispose to low back injury in gen-

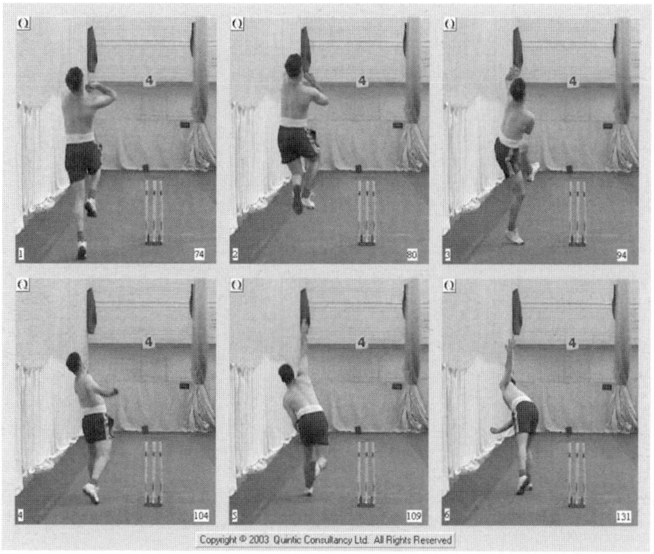

Fig. 16.5 Bowling sequence – back view. Phase 1: predelivery take-off; phase 2: mid-bound; phase 3: back-foot contact; phase 4: front-foot contact; phase 5: release; phase 6: first-foot follow-through. Reproduced with permission from Quintic Consultancy Ltd.

Table 16.4 Fast-bowlers' directives (England and Wales Cricket Board)

A. Directives for matches

Age	Maximum overs per spell	Maximum overs per day
Up to 13	4	8
U14, U15	5	10
U16, U17	6	18
U18, U19	7	21

B. Directives for practice sessions

Age	Maximum balls per session	Maximum sessions per week
Up to 13	30	2
U14, U15	36	2
U16, U17	36	3
U18, U19	42	3

eral, and spondylolysis in particular, and have been deemed faulty or dangerous. Bowling technique can be analysed by means of video analysis, and a bowler recovering from a pars stress lesion should undergo this before their return to sport (Fig. 16.5).

Bowling prescription. Table 16.4 gives the England and Wales Cricket Board (ECB) guidelines on exactly how many balls a fast bowler, of a given age, should bowl in both practice and matchplay. It is essential that players, coaches, captains and parents are made aware of these guidelines, particularly during an adolescent growth spurt.

The Australian Cricket Board (ACB) National Fast Bowling Workload and Injury Study 2000–2002 highlights the possibility of too low and infrequent a bowling workload, as well as too high a workload, as a significant risk factor, and it is the author's perception that sudden increases in bowling intensity pose a risk (just like any stress fracture), particularly in association with indoor nets on inadequately sprung surfaces.

Hand injuries in cricket

A retrospective study of finger fractures in county cricketers by Bell and Ahsan (unpublished, 2002) found that 110 cricketers reported 120 finger frac-

tures or fracture/dislocations. Fielders accounted for 46%, batsmen 39% and wicket-keepers 15%. Slip fielders are most commonly injured (14.5%), followed by midoff fielders (9%) and bowlers (5.5%). The bottom hand is vulnerable in batsmen, that is, the right hand in right-handed batsmen, and the left hand in left-handed batsmen.

The openers, number 1 and 2 batsmen, account for 30%, and the all-rounders, typically number 7 and 8 batsmen, for 31%. The nature of the game determines that the openers, and the late-middle order, often face the new ball, optionally taken by the opposition's fastest bowlers after 90 overs. The risk of finger fracture overall seems to increase with age, with players aged 32–37 accounting for 49% of finger injuries. Interestingly the fractures in cricketers are not spread around – 54% of players questioned having never sustained a finger fracture.

Splitting the webbing between the fingers is not uncommon in fielders misjudging a catch in the field – the ball forcibly abducts adjacent fingers. These should be sutured in most cases, with buddy strapping afterwards, because they have a tendency to reopen.

Knee ligament injuries

Knee ligament injuries are uncommon in cricket, but are interesting for two reasons. There have been several high-profile anterior cruciate ligament (ACL) ruptures occurring during football kickabouts used as cross-training drills, and ACL ruptures and meniscal tears can occur during the sliding stop, commonly seen in modern-day fielding practices (the author ruptured his ACL in delivery stride!).

Impingement syndromes

A number of impingement syndromes affect cricketers:

1 Posterior ankle impingement (see Chapter 8) classically affects fast bowlers, with or without associated flexor hallucis longus (FHL) tendon involvement. Usually the left ankle is affected in right-arm bowlers, occurring at front-foot impact There may be a prominent Stieda process, or an os trigonum, or simply inflamed synovium posteriorly, and the syndrome is associated with a long delivery stride, overpronation, and large foot holes.

2 Anterior ankle impingement, in association with tibial and talar osteophytes, occurs less commonly (see Chapter 8). Take great care in advocating posterior ankle surgery if the posterior impingement test is negative during clinical assessment.

3 Posterior elbow impingement is occasionally seen in fast bowlers and is intimately linked to bowling technique, affecting both the right and left elbows.

4 Shoulder impingement (see Chapter 4) is common and related to throwing rather than bowling. Once a player has 'lost their arm' it is a difficult thing to get back, with or without surgery. With the intensity of the modern one-day game it has become difficult to 'hide' one fielder, let alone two or more (a problem England were faced with in the 1996 World Cup in India and Pakistan). Take great care in advocating subacromial surgery in a bowler who can throw but cannot bowl – the last one seen by the author following failed subacromial surgery had a stress fracture of the scapula (Fig. 16.6). Suboptimal scapular stabilization, muscle imbalance with relatively weak shoulder external rotators, glenohumeral instability, as well as rusty links in the kinetic chain, are all predisposing factors (as they are in all throwing sports), and cricket has spent considerable time and energy in addressing throwing technique.

5 Impingement of the lower ribs on the iliac crest on the lead side in fast bowlers can cause considerable disability, causing the bowler to fall away in follow-through and in some cases necessitating resection of a rib. Rib stress fractures are becoming a more frequently recognized entity in fast bowlers with 'side strains', although the classical 'rib tip syndrome' (colloquially known as 'the intercostal') is most commonly due to tears of the oblique abdominals at their attachment to the free ends of the 11th and 12th ribs. It is important to consider all these entities in the differential diagnosis of chest wall pain in cricketers and to avoid the injudicious use of corticosteroid injections.

Collision with boundary fence

In first-class cricket, between 1995 and 1996, and 1999 and 2000, seven injuries occurred as a result of players colliding with the boundary fence when sliding to field the ball. This can be reduced by using a boundary rope well within the field of play and away from the advertising hoardings The author has seen small flags attached to long, thin metal stakes used as boundary markers at international matches on the Indian subcontinent (and had them removed), so it is always worth having a safety check well in advance of the start of play if you are responsible for the players' welfare.

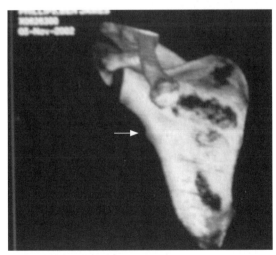

Fig. 16.6 CT of right scapula of county right-arm fast bowler with a healing stress fracture of the scapula (arrow). This bowler presented with posterior chest wall pain when bowling, but could throw. He had undergone failed subacromial decompression. Cricketers with subacromial impingement can bowl, but cannot throw!

Touring with cricket sides

Acting as physician to a cricket team on tour is a unique experience, particularly as test tours are so long. Tours of the subcontinent are particularly challenging, where the prospects of tropical illness and heat, altitude and pollution are very real. Pre-tour screening, acclimatization strategy and meticulous attention to the nutritional and hydration status of the players (take weighing scales to weigh in and out, and consider prophylactic antibiotics for a World Cup in India or Pakistan) as well as a tolerant and understanding partner at home, are crucial to your and the team's success (see Chapter 1).

Tennis

In a retrospective study of the injury experiences of adult nonelite tennis players, 44% reported an injury that prevented play in the previous 12 months. Upper and lower limb injuries were equally represented, and 72% were classified as overuse injuries. Injury to the elbow, lumbar spine, shoulder and knee were most frequently reported. This chapter describes the most common problems associated with tennis and how to deal with them.

Injury epidemiology

The above findings were borne out during a review of the epidemiological literature available. Rates of 2.3 injuries/player/1000 tennis hours are reported. Most acute injuries were classified as sprains or strains with less than 2% reflecting fracture or dislocation. The majority of chronic injuries (67%) were classified as overuse. The foot, ankle, knee, lumbar spine and shoulder are most commonly injured. Elbow injury, and in particular epicondylopathy, is typically an affliction of mature tennis players.

Injury management

The aetiology of overuse injury can be divided into factors that reflect the way we are made (intrinsic factors) and those that reflect the way we do things and the environment in which they are done (extrinsic factors) (Table 16.5). The modification of extrinsic factors is most easily achieved.

A tennis shot utilizes all components of the kinetic chain, from the racket itself, through the hand and arm and down the spine to the legs. Thus a 'problem' in one component may manifest as a symptom in another. Look beyond the presenting complaint.

Table 16.5 Overuse injury aetiology

Intrinsic factors	Extrinsic factors
Age	Technique and training errors
Gender	Environment
Biomechanics	Equipment
Height and weight	Playing surface

Specific injury problems

Shoulder problems

Tennis players are vulnerable to a number of shoulder problems including rotator cuff tendinopathy, impingement and subacromial bursitis (see Chapter 4).

Presentation

Tennis involves the coordinated interaction between the various components of the shoulder complex, which, when coupled with the sport's repetitive physical demands, can lead to overuse tendinopathy affecting the scapular stabilizers, rotator cuff and biceps. Tendinopathy will lead to weakness, affecting the coordinated function of the shoulder complex, with a progression to secondary problems, for example further loss of scapular stabilization and subacromial impingement or bursitis. Shoulder function will be affected by most of the intrinsic and extrinsic factors listed in Table 16.5; however, particular attention should be paid to technique. The effect that service action and ball toss have on the shoulder may seem obvious, but poor court position sense and/or abnormal lower body setting will leave the player wrongly positioned to execute a shot.

Symptoms will relate to the underlying pathology responsible, as mentioned above, with detailed examination confirming the diagnosis (see Chapter 4).

Management

Modification of activity and simple analgesia are the initial steps, with structured rehabilitation to strengthen rotator cuff and address scapular stability, as previously described, being a primary concern (see Chapter 4); other interventions have been detailed previously alongside the relevant pathologies. Most important, however, is the need to address any problems relating to technique or equipment, and it is here that the sports physician's knowledge and interest in sport, coupled with the multidisciplinary approach that encourages working alongside coaches, etc., becomes important.

Faults that may cause injury include:
• Inadequate knee bend and an inability to transfer force from legs through the arm during the tennis serve, increases the demands on the shoulder to create service speed, placing the shoulder at risk of injury.

• Poorly placed ball toss may result in excessive spinal extension and encourage shoulder impingement.

• Poor court positioning increases the likelihood of incorrect ground-stroke action, which may result in shoulder injury.

Elbow problems
Presentation

Tennis elbow (lateral epicondylitis/epicondylosis) is the classical elbow complaint and may be present either acutely as an enthesitis or more often as a more chronic tendinopathy at the common wrist extensor origin, and in particular the extensor carpi radialis brevis (ECRB) (see Chapter 5).

Many factors have been identified as increasing the risk of occurrence, primarily age (usually mature players >35 in the case of tendinopathy), improper grip size, excessive racket head vibration (tight strings, heavy racket), poor backhand technique (snapping wrist) and high-intensity play.

Management

Acute management comprises the usual modalities of ice post-exercise and NSAIDs.

Rehabilitation then consists of soft tissue techniques to help in symptom resolution, concentrating on improving wrist extensor flexibility, alongside an intensive eccentric strengthening programme. Counter braces seem to help some players, whilst steroid injections are occasionally used in difficult cases. Importantly the predisposing factors mentioned earlier should be addressed to prevent recurrence.

Tennis leg: medial gastrocnemius strain
Presentation

Tennis leg reflects a muscle strain or tear to the medial head of gastrocnemius. The gastrocnemius is one of a number of muscles that cross two joints, in this case the knee and ankle. It takes origin from the medial and lateral posterior femoral condyles/distal femur and joins with soleus to form the Achilles tendon. It therefore flexes the knee and plantarflexes the foot.

All such muscles are prone to injury because of their unusual requirement to work both eccentrically and concentrically. It has been suggested that other factors such as tibialis anterior/gastrocnemius muscle imbalance or excessive pronation, are also contributory.

The history is usually one of sudden discomfort in the calf, often occurring when jumping for a shot. Palpation reveals discomfort around the medial head of the gastrocnemius, exacerbated by resisted plantarflexion and passive dorsiflexion.

Management

Initial management consists of RICE (rest, ice, compression, elevation) to minimize further damage, followed by a structured course of rehabilitation, consisting of an eccentric exercise programme and intensive soft tissue work, often including ischaemic massage techniques. An assessment of lower limb biomechanics should be undertaken and corrections made if indicated.

Tennis toe (subungal haematoma)
Presentation

This condition usually affects the big toe nail (occasionally the second if longer) and is the result of traumatic swelling and bleeding underneath the nail, the lateral side being more often affected. The cause is modern tennis shoes, designed to maximize grip. Repeated sudden stops force the foot to slide within the shoe, and unless there is sufficient space, the nail is jammed into the shoe.

Management

Avoidance is better than cure, with correct shoe fitting and regular trimming of toe nails. Cold packs are used to reduce swelling alongside adequate analgesia. Felt padding to the base of the nail may reduce discomfort during play. Subungal haematomas may require release, via a hole in the nail. An extensive haematoma (>25%) might indicate an underlying fracture.

Lumbar spine problems
Presentation

The spine can be divided into three columns: anterior, middle and posterior. The posterior column incorporates the pars interarticularis (the thin cortical bony connection between the pedicle and lamina), the facet joints and the spinous process. Normally the facet joints bear approximately 20% of the compressive spinal load; however, this increases during extension and unilaterally in rotation to the ipsilateral side.

The tennis serve involves repetitive lumbar spinal extension and rotation and therefore excessive loading of the posterior column. This stress is potentiated by poor service action and a backward ball throw. The resultant repetitive loading may lead to either a stress fracture of the pars interarticularis (most commonly at L5) or facet joint injury, characterized by hypomobility (synovitis, capsular shortening and fibrosis) or hypermobility (capsular laxity). Examination usually reveals localized tenderness to palpation with discomfort being reproduced on hyperextension and rotation to the affected side. Failure to recognize a pars stress fracture and reduce excessive overload may lead to progression to a true pars defect (spondylolysis). When a spondylolysis is associated with instability (forward slippage of the superior vertebra) the term spondylolisthesis is used.

Pars defects may also reflect a genetic fibrous pseudoarthrosis (5% of children over 7 years of age). Thus the presence of a pars defect does not necessarily imply traumatic overload, and equally may not be the explanation for back pain. Concordance between mechanism of injury, clinical evaluation and imaging studies is necessary to confirm the diagnosis.

Further investigation and management follow the principles described earlier (see under 'Cricket' above), with the highlighting and correction of any technical factors that may be causative, being essential.

Tennis is a wonderful game. It requires aerobic fitness, teamwork and mental agility. Although serious injury is extremely unlikely, acute and chronic soft tissue overuse injuries may occur. An understanding of the likely injuries and their aetiology will help firstly to prevent injury and secondly to ensure an early return to the sport.

Further reading

Carroll R. Tennis elbow: incidence in local league players. *Br J Sports Med* 1981, **15,** 250–256.

Feit EM, Berenter R. Lower extremity tennis injuries. Prevalence, aetiology and mechanism. *J Am Podiatr Med Assoc* 1993, **83,** 509–515.

Kamien M. The incidence of tennis elbow and other injuries in tennis players at the Royal Kings Park Tennis Club of Western Australia from October 1983 to September 1984. *Aust J Sci Med Sport* 1989, **6,** 18–22.

Lawn Tennis Association, www.lta.org.uk

Moore KL. *Clinically Orientated Anatomy,* 3rd edn. Baltimore, Williams & Wilkins, 1992.

Physician and Sports Medicine, www.physsportsmed.com

Reid DC. *Sports Injury Assessment and Rehabilitation,* 1st edn. New York, Churchill Livingstone, 1992.

Sandor RS, Brone S. Rehabilitating ankle sprains. *Physician and Sports Med* 2002, **30,** 48–50.

Winge S, Jorgenson U, Nielson L. Epidemiology of injuries in Danish championship tennis. *Int J Sports Med* 1989, **10,** 368–371.

Skiing and snowboarding

Alpine skiing and snowboarding are amongst the most popular of winter sports. Whilst skiing is a long-established sport, snowboarding has dramatically increased in popularity over the last 15 years. In the USA, in the 1999–2000 season, there were over 52 million skiing days (one skiing day is one visit to a ski resort by a skier or a snowboarder).

Although both sports are practised on the same slopes, the pattern of injuries associated with each sport is different. The average skier is aged 31, and 60% are male. The average snowboarder is aged 20 and 75% are male. The overall injury rate is between 3 and 4.5 injuries per 1000 skiing days.

Skiing

Improper maintenance and adjustment of equipment is responsible for 44% of all downhill ski injuries. In skiing, the high speeds achieved by the skier engender large forces applied to the unnaturally lengthened foot by the ski-binding/boot system, resulting in significant injury, particularly to the lower limb. As many as 30% of all ski injuries probably result from failure of the ski binding to function properly.

Snowboarding

Salient statistics here are that 36% of those injured have never snowboarded before, and 25% are in their first year of snowboarding. Wrist injuries predominate in the beginner group (41%), whereas it is the shoulder in intermediates (38%) and head injuries in experts (36%). The average distribution of snowboarding injuries is:

- Wrist   23%
- Ankle   16%
- Knee   16%
- Head   9%
- Shoulder   8%
- Other   28%.

Anterior shoulder dislocation

Presentation

Anterior shoulder dislocations represent about 30% of ski and snowboarding-related shoulder injuries. This injury occurs mainly from falling backwards onto an outstretched arm. The force of the fall on the ground pushes the arm forwards causing the shoulder to dislocate anteriorly (see Chapter 4). Alternatively, if one of the ski poles gets stuck in the snow, the shoulder can be pushed forwards, causing it again to dislocate anteriorly. Observation reveals the characteristic deformity of the shoulder, with a prominent humeral head and a hollow below the acromion, which in association with the history and other symptomatology, usually makes the diagnosis obvious. Further investigation, to exclude associated injuries, and management are detailed in Chapter 4. This is an injury that carries a high rate of recurrence in the young sportsperson and so correct rehabilitation and management is vital.

Fractured wrist

Presentation

As documented previously, the wrist is the most common site of injury in skiing and snowboarding, making up nearly a quarter (23%) of all injuries and half of all fractures. The most frequently fractured carpal bone is the scaphoid. (Other carpal fractures include those of the triquetral and hook of hamate.)

Falling backwards is the mechanism in 75% of wrist injuries, usually with the wrist bent backwards on an extended arm. Moderate pain is felt, with reduction in power of the hand movements. There is swelling in the scaphoid region and tenderness in the 'anatomical snuff box' (see Chapter 5).

Management

X-rays should include a 'scaphoid view' (postero-anterior in ulnar deviation) but may be negative. If so, place the wrist in a 'scaphoid cast' and re-X-ray at 2 weeks. (Remember that nonunion, and/or avascular necrosis of the proximal fragment may occur, particularly if the fracture is missed.) If a fracture is present, immobilize in a plaster cast for a minimum of 8 weeks (12 weeks is the median time for union). Fractures demonstrating greater than 2 mm displacement should proceed straight to open reduction and internal fixation (ORIF).

Ulnar collateral ligament thumb injury

Presentation

Known as 'skier's thumb' or 'gamekeeper's thumb', this is the most commonly occurring upper limb injury in skiers, and comprises 7% of all skiing injuries. The mechanism is one of the skier falling onto an outstretched arm, and in so doing, forcing the thumb upwards (abduction) and backwards (extension) against the ski pole. Examination will reveal bruising, swelling and pain in the thumb web space, with tenderness to palpation over the ulnar aspect of the metacarpophalangeal (MCP) joint. Instability of the joint is demonstrated when the thumb is tested in abduction at an angle of 20–30° – critical laxity (indicating total rupture) being 30° greater than the normal opposite thumb.

Management

An X-ray may demonstrate bony avulsion of the ulnar side of the proximal phalanx. Stress films may identify complete tears with Stener's lesions (adductor aponeurosis interposition). Grade of injury determines treatment:
- Types I (sprain) and II (partial tear) – splint for 6 weeks in thumb spica or S-Thumb splint.
- Type III (complete tear with >30° abduction possible) – surgical repair is advocated.

Anterior cruciate ligament rupture

Presentation

Anterior cruciate ligament (ACL) injuries have tripled since the late 1970s and make up 33% of all skiing-associated knee injuries. Two mechanisms are identified. The first involves the skier falling backwards on landing, the rear of the ski striking the snow and the boot producing an anterior draw loading to the proximal tibia. As the foot is driven flat on the snow the ACL is disrupted.

The second is an uncontrolled fall with the skier falling backwards, resulting in the rear of the ski carving a turn, producing internal rotation of the tibia as the knee flexes past 90°. This can produce an isolated injury to the ACL but might also damage the posterolateral components of the knee. Combination injuries involving the collateral ligaments and menisci are common. Further symptoms and signs accompanying this injury are described in Chapter 7, along with a management plan.

Tibial fracture

Presentation

Lower leg fracture remains the third most common injury seen among alpine skiers. Snow conditions are an important consideration in tibial fractures – on icy or hard-packed surfaces the incidence of tibial fractures is much lower than in powder snow.

A fall in any direction may result in the lever action of the ski greatly increasing the rotational forces applied to the tibia, resulting in fracture. Activities such as landing awkwardly from jumps or turns may similarly incur injury.

Injury causes intense pain at the site of the fracture with tenderness and swelling locally. Inability to weight bear may be secondary to displacement of the fracture with loss of contour and alignment of the lower leg. Fracture of the tibia is often compound and visible through the damaged skin.

Management

Circulatory and neurological status distal to the injury should be rapidly assessed. X-rays will identify the nature and extent of the bony injury. Most closed tibial fractures can be treated conservatively, as long as angulation is minimal, with an above-knee plaster keeping the knee slightly flexed and the ankle in 90° of dorsiflexion. Displaced and compound fractures require operative repair. Bony union requires 8–12 weeks or sometimes longer. Physiotherapy after removal of the plaster is aimed at restoring strength and range of movement in both knee and ankle.

Ankle/foot fractures

Presentation

Ankle and foot fractures are now predominantly seen in snowboarders. Fifty percent of ankle injuries are fractures. These may be classified using a variety of schemes depending on the components involved (e.g. Weber's, Henderson's, Launge-Hansen). Osteochondral fracture of the talar dome or lateral process of the talus may be overlooked. The flexibility of the snowboarding boot allows the foot/ankle complex to be traumatized in all directions, depending on the nature of the fall. Symptoms and signs will usually be significant enough to suggest an underlying fracture, with weightbearing often proving difficult and X-ray confirming suspicions.

Management

Undisplaced fractures in association with a stable joint require immobilization in plaster cast or ankle brace for 4–8 weeks. Unstable ankles and displaced fractures require open reduction and internal fixation. Rehabilitation depends on the nature of the injury and the duration of immobilization, but will include range of movement and strengthening exercises, along with proprioceptive training at an early stage.

Further reading

Abu-Laban RB. Snowboarding injuries: an analysis and comparison with alpine skiing injuries. *Can Med Assoc J* 1991, **145,** 1097–1103.

Bruckner P, Khan K. *Clinical Sports Medicine.* Sydney, McGraw Hill, 2000.

Macnab A, Cadman R. Demographics of alpine skiing and snowboarding injury: lessons for prevention programs. *Injury Prevention* 1996, **2,** 286–289.

Oxford Textbook of Sports Medicine, 2nd edn. Oxford Medical Publications, 1998.

Peterson L, Renström P. *Sports Injuries. Their Prevention and Treatment,* 3rd edn. London, Martin Dunitz, 2002.

Sutherland A, Holmes J, Myers S. Differing injury patterns in snowboarding and alpine skiing. *Injury* 1996, **27,** 423–425.

17 Drugs in sport

Sporting headlines that are newsworthy contain controversy as often as they report achievement. The abuse of drugs in sport can be traced back as far as the ancient Greeks, when their Olympians experimented with various naturally occurring remedies, in an attempt to improve performance by using their stimulating properties.

Cycling features prominently as a sport with problems, and this is not confined to the modern era. Stories date back to the end of the 19th century, with competitors in the Tour de France catching trains and taking short cuts to gain an advantage, these methods being eclipsed by the use of highly toxic concoctions of caffeine, strychnine (in high doses a commonly chosen lethal poison of the era) and cocaine.

Amphetamines became the drug of choice in the 1950s, often precipitating collapse as cyclists exceeded their physiological capabilities, with some unfortunate fatalities. Marathon runners used similar methods, with high-dose caffeine ingestion having been noted even in recent times, before the classification of caffeine as a restricted substance, illegal above a stated level (now removed).

The sports physician must remain up to date with all changes that occur in the list of banned substances, enabling them to give accurate, informed advice on what is and is not legal for the athlete. Ignorance is no excuse and all too often an unfortunate competitor has fallen foul either as a result of their own failure to ask for advice or occasionally as a result of their team physician's misinformation. Surprisingly, mistakes still occur at the highest level. Recent Olympic Games have produced a number of such incidents, causing innocent competitors to lose their placing and any medal, and sometimes face lengthy bans from their sport, following the use of seemingly innocuous substances such as simple cold remedies. With positive tests also having apparently arisen following the use of contaminated supplements, advice must clearly state that the athlete is responsible for all substances they ingest, whether as medicines or supplements.

High-profile cases have led to scepticism among the public about the validity of records or levels of performance in certain sports. This alone is a valid argument to put to those who might question the continual pursuit of drug-free competition.

The IOC Medical Code

The standard classification of prohibited and restricted substances drawn up by the International Olympic Committee (IOC) is now widely used in sport, and is summarized here. There are three classes:

Class I – Prohibited classes of substances
Class II – Prohibited methods
Class III – Classes of drugs subject to restriction.

A comprehensive list of all substances within these classes can be found on the UK Sport website, given at the end of the chapter. The discussion below details the more commonly encountered drugs that are abused either intentionally or in ignorance, the latter excuse unfortunately holding no water as a defence.

Class I: prohibited classes of substances

Prohibited substances are divided into the following pharmacological categories:
- stimulants;
- narcotics;
- anabolic agents;

- diuretics;
- peptide hormones.

Stimulants

Substances taken by many on a daily basis that until recently fell within this category were caffeine, pseudoephedrine and salbutamol. Caffeine's origins require no further explanation and a recorded level >12 µg/mL constituted a positive result up until December 2003. In real terms this equated to the equivalent of approximately six cups of strong coffee drunk during the 2 hours before competition. This would have been unlikely before most sports as it would have left the competitor running to the toilet rather than for the ball.

Pseudoephedrine is a constituent in many of the products designed to produce symptomatic relief of cold symptoms. Usually ingested in innocence, there was, as with caffeine, a threshold. This fairly innocuous medicine, the cause of many lost medals and blighted careers, was removed from the banned substance list in December 2003.

Rules regarding the use of salbutamol and other β_2-agonists have been subject to a number of changes over the last few years, with stringent restrictions now having been imposed on its use even in the inhaled form. New rulings demand that the use of salbutamol by any competitor is not only notified to the relevant governing body, but that the diagnosis of asthma or exercise-induced asthma is confirmed by 'properly qualified medical personnel' (defined as a respiratory specialist or national governing body medical officer). The IOC and certain other sports also demand that the athlete has further to show one of the following:
- a positive bronchodilator test, i.e. at least 15% increase in FEV_1 after bronchodilator use; or
- a positive bronchial provocation test (i.e. exercise test or EVH – eucapnic voluntary hyperpnoea), which is 'a fall of at least 10% in FEV_1 within 30 min of ceasing challenge'; or
- a positive bronchoconstrictor test, defined as a fall of 15% or more in FEV_1 after inhalation of a hypertonic aerosol (e.g. 4.5% saline).

These results must be notified to the relevant governing body, for example the International Amateur Athletics Federation (IAAF) in the case of athletics, by completing an abbreviated TUE (Therapeutic Use Exemption) form.

These changes have brought with them much controversy, and one must question the reasoning or lack of it behind the previous inclusion of the first two now legal substances, and more significantly the recent increased restrictions placed on salbutamol, a substance that in the inhaled form will undoubtedly produce a tremor and tachycardia when taken to excess, effects that can hardly be deemed performance enhancing.

The abuse of amphetamines dates back at least to the 1950s, as previously mentioned, when they were a common choice of the endurance cyclist. High-profile stories of their use were also reported through the 1970s and 80s within sports ranging from athletics to football.

Cocaine is banned, although its usefulness in modern day professional sport is questionable, despite its prevalence in the early 1990s. Positives tend to arise as a result of its recreational use, rather than its being taken for its performance-enhancing effects.

Narcotics

Potent medications in this group, such as diamorphine and pethidine, are banned; both significantly increase pain thresholds and also produce a euphoric sense of invincibility. Medications such as codeine and dextropropoxyphene are now fortunately allowed, sparing the previously embarrassing situations where the innocent athlete is banned after consuming an analgesic only a step up from paracetamol, with no real performance-enhancing capabilities whatsoever.

Anabolic agents

Anabolic steroid use epitomizes, to the layperson, the whole issue of drug abuse in sport, often producing front page news. The effect of such drugs is one of tissue building, increasing muscle mass whilst having a positive affect on LBM (lean body mass). One of the ways they appear to facilitate this is by allowing the athlete to train 'harder and longer'.

Immediate side effects such as acne and increased aggression (the 'rugoid rage') alongside increased sexual appetite may be noticed, with long-term effects such as sterility, liver tumours, cardiomyopathies, coronary heart disease and renal failure unfortunately claiming lives long after the clamour of athletic achievements has subsided.

Testosterone has been abused for many years, with evidence of systematic use having come to light since the end of the 'cold war'. Detection relies on the measurement of the testosterone/epitestosterone ratio, which if greater than 6:1 is indicative of abuse.

More recently nandrolone (19-nortestosterone) has made the headlines, with a number of high-profile sportsmen having tested positive for its use. The metabolite 19-norandrosterone is the substance measured, its presence occurring for a number of reasons. Firstly, it has been found that nandrolone is naturally produced in small amounts in some individuals, whilst other substances, such as norethisterone, also produce the same metabolite. The amounts, however, are small and documentation before testing should avoid confusion. For this reason a positive result is only recorded for levels above 2 ng/mL in males or 5 ng/mL in females.

Some have blamed certain food supplements as being responsible for positive results. However, there is no evidence to support this claim. The only suggestions made following a review by UK Sport were that some nutritional supplements may contain steroids either intentionally or inadvertently and that boar and horse offal should be avoided as it may contain higher than normal amounts of nandrolone.

Finasteride, a 5-alpha-reductase inhibitor, will reduce the excretion of the metabolite and can be used to mask its use; however, it is not as yet on the banned list.

β_2-Agonists are also included in this group, with one study reporting that clenbuterol has an anabolic effect. For this reason they are prohibited both via the oral and injectable route, being allowed only in the inhaled preparation, with even this method of administration being rigidly restricted as stated above. A level of salbutamol >1000 ng/mL is deemed a positive result.

Diuretics

Bumetanide and frusemide are examples of drugs within this category that are abused in two ways. In the first instance they may be used to help reduce

weight, a tactic sometimes employed in sports such as judo or boxing, where eligibility to compete within a certain category is dependent on achieving the required weight. A further use of this category of drugs is to dilute urine, in an attempt to mask the excretion of certain substances.

Reported findings seem to be less common now as more sophisticated methods of pharmaceutical manipulation seem to be favoured.

Peptide hormones

Corticotropins (e.g. adrenocorticotropic hormone, ACTH), human chorionic gonadotropin (HCG: males only), growth hormone (hGH) and pituitary gonadotropins (e.g. luteinizing hormone, LH: males only) are examples within this group. They are used for their anabolic effect on muscle, improved tissue healing and positive effect on lean body mass. Abuse of these substances is unfortunately widespread, despite the potential risks of developing illnesses ranging from diabetes to colorectal cancer or breast cancer. Due to their natural occurrence, detection is particularly difficult.

EPO (erythropoietin) also falls within this group. It is used to artificially increase red cell production and therefore oxygen-carrying capacity of the blood. Its prevalence has been widely publicized both in cycling, a sport in which it has been abused for well over a decade, and in distance running. A combination of blood and urine tests is now available for detection, and was first put into practice at the Sydney Olympics. Cycling takes a slightly different approach. Following a number of deaths from cardiac or cerebral thrombosis due to the hyperviscosity resulting from its use, it was decided to ban competitors from competing if blood testing before an event reveals a packed cell volume (PCV) above a level considered to be medically inadvisable.

Unfortunately there are always those who remain one step ahead of the game, and reliable sources have recounted incidences of competitors retiring to bed with an intravenous (i.v.) line in situ, having already checked their PCV using their own portable haematocrit. This enables them to manipulate the result with i.v. fluids should they be woken with a knock on the door signalling an early morning pre-race blood test.

Insulin is also included in this group, and is only allowed in those who have been medically certified as suffering with insulin-dependent diabetes.

Class II: prohibited methods

There are several categories of prohibited methods:
• blood doping;
• manipulation;
• pharmaceutical;
• chemical;
• physical.

Blood doping

Blood doping is the practice whereby an individual augments his or her own red cell pool with an infusion of either whole blood or packed cells. The blood used is removed from the athlete some months earlier, at a time when peak performance is not required, and is then stored. It is reinfused some months later when the athlete has naturally replaced their circulating volume. The idea is to increase red cell volume and as a consequence artificially increase oxygen-carrying capacity.

Although common in the 1970s and 1980s, its use has declined with the advent of the above-mentioned more complex methods, although it is still used because it is almost undetectable.

Manipulation

Manipulation of a sample includes the use, as mentioned above, of masking drugs such as diuretics and probenecid, that will increase excretion rates and therefore clearance of a banned substance.

Athletes have even been found with 'clean' urine in the bladder obtained from other sources and instilled via self-catheterization. One such competitor inadvertently incriminated themselves when the sample showed the presence of a contraceptive hormone; this would not in itself have been a problem had the competitor in question not been male.

Testosterone detection can be masked by the additional ingestion of epitestosterone in an attempt at maintaining the testosterone/epitestosterone ratio whilst abusing the former.

Attempts to alter the integrity or validity of a sample are viewed as illegal whether successful or not.

Class III: restricted substances

Alcohol is subject to various restrictions, with individual authorities operating within their own jurisdiction as to the level of punishment for a positive test. The Football Association, for example, will refer the result to the club medical officer, sensible in that alcohol abuse often harms only the user. This approach allows the individual to seek the necessary help.

Cannabinoids, a recreational drug, again are subject to individual jurisdiction, with the IOC deeming a urinary concentration of its metabolite greater than 15 ng/mL as positive for doping.

Local anaesthetics are allowed if medically justified either as local or intra-articular injection, but their use must be notified to the governing bodies. Adrenaline (epinephrine) is permitted with these local injections.

Corticosteroids are allowable via all routes other than oral, rectal, intravenous or intramuscular. Their use, however, either via the inhaled or injectable route (intra-articular or local) needs to be notified to the necessary governing body via the completion of an abbreviated TUE (topical use no longer requires notification).

Beta-blockers are prohibited by certain sports, such as archery, diving, shooting, gymnastics, fencing and equestrian pursuits, where a clear advantage could be gained by their effect in reducing tremor.

Restrictions regarding the use of asthma medication have been dealt with above.

Other groups

Supplements such as creatine and Actovegin are now under close scrutiny. Studies testing the purity of creatine supplements have demonstrated that this preparation from certain companies contained nandrolone. Whether its presence was intentional, to augment the anabolic effect (one of the legal aims of creatine) or unintentional as a result of contamination during production, is unclear.

The overall advice to athletes regarding supplements should be that most of the benefits claimed are unproven and are unnecessary in those on a balanced diet. Extra care should be taken regarding foreign and herbal medicines, as the exact contents are often unclear.

Summary

In summary, the athlete should be advised to question any medication or supplement that they are taking, and if in doubt professional advice should be sought.

Detailed information, both for the clinician or athlete, can be accessed through the websites given under 'Further reading'.

Further reading

UK Sport, www.uksport.gov.uk
World Anti-Doping Agency, www.wada-ama.org

18 Concepts in rehabilitation

The term 'rehabilitation' refers to the process of restoring normal function following injury. Rehabilitation of the injured athlete begins immediately following the injury. Prompt and appropriate intervention aims to optimize an athlete's return to training and competition.

Rehabilitation is a broad concept that requires the clinician to draw on an extensive knowledge base. This includes an understanding of:

- tissue response to injury;
- the adaptive response of tissue to load;
- the load demands of the sport or activity, including the causes or mechanisms of injury, e.g. biomechanical;
- clinical ability and techniques to alter these causal factors;
- structuring a rehabilitation programme to consider a wide range of factors;
- return to sport (RTS) – where does the rehab finish and the training begin?

Using the evidence to build the case

Rehabilitation, by its nature, is subjective and individualized. Whilst ongoing research adds to our knowledge base, it should be noted that often there is little evidence in the literature to support the techniques and approaches we employ in physical therapies within sport.

Anecdotally, many of the techniques employed appear to be effective. However, with the continual push towards evidence-based medicine, there is the expectation that these techniques are in fact reliably effective. On the other hand, one has to consider the many limitations that accompany research involving elite athletes. It is up to the therapist to weigh the literary evidence (and methodology) against the population base they are treating and the results they are achieving and so decide the best course of action.

In essence, the therapist should engage in reflective practice wherever possible, remain up to date with the current literature, reflect on the results achieved, and tailor the rehabilitation programme to the individual.

Tissue response to injury

What happens post-injury?

Immediately post-injury there is disruption of the normal structure and function of the tissues. Pain and inflammation will produce a response leading rapidly to muscle inhibition and atrophy. These effects must be minimized in the first instance, before any specific intervention is undertaken.

Acute management

Rehabilitation should begin as soon as injury occurs. The use of RICE (rest, ice, compression and elevation) to control pain and inflammation is common in an attempt to minimize secondary hypoxic cell damage.

The goal of early stage rehabilitation is to restore function as soon as possible. Combining the effects of stretching, strengthening and neural patterning with other techniques in the therapist's arsenal should be used to achieve optimal function.

The adaptive response of tissue to load

A basic understanding of the response to conditioning in muscle, tendon and bone is essential to those involved in rehabilitation.

Muscle

Muscle, like most tissues, will respond to mechanical loading, resulting in an increase in strength. This is the basic premise behind strengthening the musculoskeletal system and is known as 'specific adaptation to imposed demand' (SAID). Once the tissues have adapted to this stimulus then further adaptation can be brought about by altering the intensity, speed, duration, volume, range, frequency, type, recovery period, function or specificity of the exercise.

Excessive loading, however, may be counterproductive, resulting in tissue breakdown. Therefore it is the clinician's ability to design a training programme resulting in the appropriate recruitment of the appropriate motor units in a functionally correct way that will lead to the desired result.

Tendon

Tendon is noncontractile connective tissue that transfers the force produced by muscle to the bone, thereby producing movement. It is an area that is often injured, with common sites including the Achilles and patellar tendons. The method of injury and the process of repair are poorly understood. As such, tendon injuries are often resistant to treatment, posing a significant challenge to their management. Intervention is often based on clinical experience, with the management of an Achilles tendinopathy being given as an example later in this chapter.

Bone

Bone disruption will occur when load exceeds strength, either acutely as a traumatic fracture, or following the application of repeated low-level loads, resulting in a stress fracture.

The causation of stress fractures is often multifactorial. An increased biomechanical stress, such as excessive pronation, is one cause. Equally, sudden alterations in training load, intensity, frequency or volume can lead to bone breakdown. Inappropriate footwear or training surface are also factors, the simple suggestion of updating footwear regularly

sometimes being all that is necessary to avoid recurrences of stress fractures.

Clinical ability and techniques to alter causal factors

Once the initial phase has been managed, a differential diagnosis has been established, and the causal factors are recognized and addressed, the therapist must institute a rehabilitation management plan. The following factors should be addressed:
- instituting pain-free movement;
- strength of the muscle-tendon unit;
- flexibility;
- proprioception;
- core strength/stability;
- functional retraining of movement;
- taping to reduce pain or to limit (or facilitate) movement;
- cross-training to maintain cardiovascular fitness;
- psychological factors.

Instituting pain-free movement

Of the many tools the therapist has available, electrotherapy has traditionally been used to achieve initial functional pain-free movement, despite little evidence that many of the modalities used actually do what many claim. The therapist is encouraged to continually assess the role of electrotherapy in the rehabilitation process.

Manual therapy plays a major part. Mobilization of tight structures to facilitate movement patterns and increase joint range and mobility are areas that therapists describe as being integral to achieving the desired result.

Strength of the muscle-tendon unit

Strength training will increase the size and strength of the muscle-tendon unit. The benefits to the rehabilitation process are obvious.

Progressive loading of the musculoskeletal system involves applying stimuli and allowing adaptation, before applying a slightly larger stimulus. Changing the intensity, duration, volume, frequency, rest intervals or exercise type can vary the load. The type of exercise may include free weights, resistance machines, body-weight or elastic bands (theraband). Varying the training method, between isometric, isokinetic, eccentric and plyometric loading, can also be incorporated.

A correctly designed strength-training programme will produce significant benefits, but it must be specific to the patient. A power event athlete would not need a high degree of endurance-based work, especially towards the end of the rehabilitation phase, and so the knowledge and experience of the coach need to be utilized and considered.

'Strength and conditioning', in the elite sports performer, has become a specialist field. The clinician needs to become familiar with the broad concept, but as with all paramedical and medical areas, should develop a close working relationship with the strength and conditioning service provider.

Flexibility

As with the rest of the rehabilitation programme, the role of flexibility must be assessed on an individual basis. Regaining full flexibility of joints, muscles and other tissues, bearing in mind the requirements of the sport, is an essential part of the rehabilitation process. Lack of flexibility in key areas may actually have contributed to the original injury. That said, there is currently little conclusive evidence in the literature supporting the use of stretching in an attempt to decrease the number, frequency or severity of injury. As with all aspects of the rehabilitation process, a holistic approach should be taken, with firm rationale behind each stage of the process.

As an example, we could take the incidence of hamstring strains. Research has suggested that flexibility of the hamstring is no indication as to whether an athlete will or will not sustain a hamstring injury. Research has also suggested that restricted hip extension causes the pelvis to rotate anteriorly, producing increased movement of the lumbar spine. If the premise is that many hamstring strains are related to adverse neural mechanics, then it may be that these anterior structures should be included within a stretching programme, ensuring adequate flexibility around the front of the hip, and facilitating more effective lumbar spine mechanics.

Basic guidelines for the types of stretching or mobility work that will improve joint or muscle ranges include:

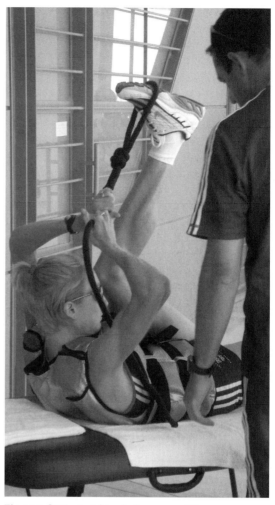

Fig. 18.1 Static stretching before competition.

Static (Fig. 18.1):
- most popular and widely known;
- relatively safe;
- no partner needed;
- passive stretching of a specific muscle by placing it on maximum stretch and holding it for a nominated period of time;
- time may vary from 3 to 60+ seconds;
- number of repetitions and frequency per day can be individualized.

Dynamic/ballistic:
- repetitive contractions of the agonist muscle are used to produce quick stretches of the antagonist muscle;

• needs to be controlled and has potential to cause injury;

• should only be used by experienced athletes;

• often used after static stretching and can be tailored to more dynamic (sport-specific) activities.

PNF (proprioceptive neuromuscular facilitation):

• based on neurophysiological principles;

• contract–relax and hold–relax;

• approximately 10–15-second hold;

• agonist is contracted near end of range; muscle is then taken further into range during relaxation phase;

• generally requires a partner;

• both athlete and partner should be experienced and should not force the body part beyond comfortable range.

General principles for safe stretching include:

• Gradual progression into the stretch.

• Stretching should be controlled and never forced into end range.

• Hold time will be individualized. Research is ongoing looking at the length of the stretch as applied to performance, and appears to be indicating a direction of a combination of short active stretches.

• Individualize stretches to the athlete and the event/sport.

Core strength and motor patterning

The term 'core stability' has received a lot of attention in recent years. Studies have shown a functional differentiation of the activation patterns of the abdominal musculature in exercise. The role of the deep abdominal musculature, such as transversus abdominis (TA), is integral in providing intersegmental stability of the lumbar spine. The TA is the deepest of the abdominal muscles and attaches to the lumbar spine via thoracolumbar fascia. It is through this mechanism that the TA provides intersegmental stability. Ongoing research indicates that TA function is compromised in subjects with lower back pain. Normal function must be regained to achieve a successful rehabilitation outcome.

What remains controversial is the role and recruitment patterns of the more global abdominal musculature, such as the obliques and rectus abdominis, during higher level functional activities. Research is ongoing, but it appears that the role of all these muscles (both global and intersegmental) alters significantly at higher levels of function; these current concepts should be appropriately integrated into the rehabilitation/strength programme of the elite athlete. It should not be forgotten that although the high-level athlete trains for a designated number of hours a day, for the rest of the time he or she is as sedentary as the normal population. It is likely that athletes with a history of lower back pain/dysfunction will have poor recruitment patterns of their intersegmental stabilizers. Conversely, it is probable that the athlete without a history of lower back pain will not have poor recruitment patterns.

There are many methods employed in producing core stability and core strength in the athlete, some examples being the use of Swiss Balls, Pilates and other exercise programmes. These approaches are constantly changing and so the choice is up to the individual practitioner.

Taping

Taping can be used as an adjunct to rehabilitation. The role of taping can be to:

• Decrease pain.

• Offload structures following injury.

• Limit movement of a specific joint or body part.

• Allow movement of a specific joint or body part.

• Provide proprioceptive or sensory feedback to facilitate rehabilitation.

Taping does not replace the need to undergo a strengthening or control programme. Care should also be taken, as incorrectly applied taping may aggravate an existing condition or even cause a new injury.

Guidelines for taping

• Skin preparation (clean, dry and preferably shaved well before taping).

• Dress any cuts or broken skin before applying tape.

• Use tape adherent if required.

• Use underwrap if the athlete is hyperallergic.

• Select appropriate sized tape.

• Place joint in desired position.

• Start taping with anchor piece.

• If taping over muscle, allow for expansion of the area.

- Overlap the tape and ensure no wrinkles or gaps.
- Ensure even tension of the tape and contour to the area.
- Finish with a locking piece.

After taping, ensure there is no impairment of circulation or sensation. Gain feedback from the athlete to ensure the tape is not too tight. Check to see that the tape is doing the job it was intended to do (i.e. decreasing pain, limiting range, etc.; Fig. 18.2).

The effectiveness of taping will decrease as exercise duration increases. The length of time that taping remains effective is controversial.

When removing the tape, use blunt nose scissors or a tape cutter. Pull the tape off slowly (see Chapter 7).

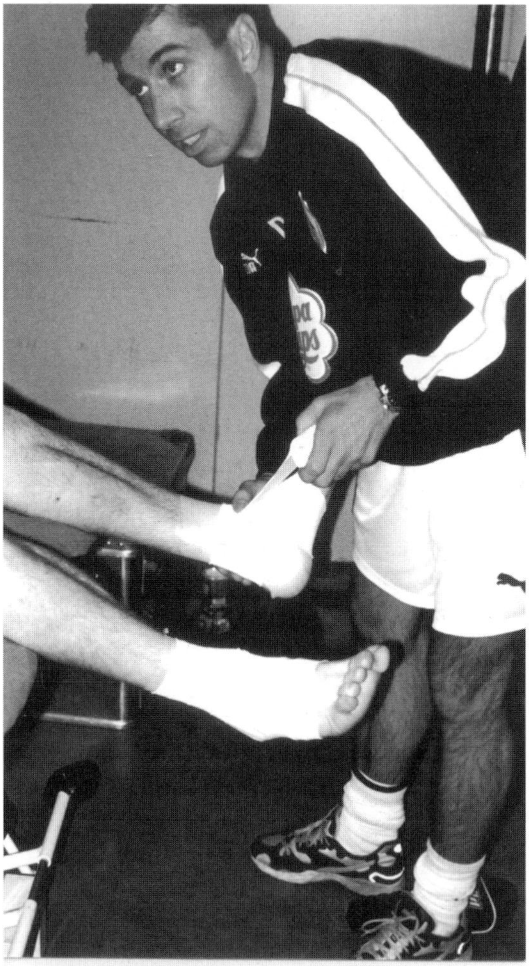

Fig. 18.2 Ankle taping.

Structuring a rehabilitation programme to consider a wide range of factors

Individualizing a programme to improve compliance

Rehabilitation should not be 'recipe book' in its approach. Each injury will have a slightly different presentation. It is important that the individual needs of the athlete are considered in the rehabilitation process. Time spent educating the athlete about the nature of the problem, the direction of the treatment regimes and possible complications, will assist in motivation and compliance. There needs to be flexibility in the programme relating to 'rate of progress'. Complications must be identified early and dealt with appropriately.

Goal orientated and restoration of function

Rehabilitation should be goal-orientated, with elite athletic performance in mind. The use of cross-training within the process allows the athlete to return to competition having lost the minimum of fitness. Too often, the rehabilitation focuses on restoring function to a specific body part, with the athlete and practitioner neglecting other areas such as flexibility, cardiovascular fitness, core strength, and strength and conditioning of other muscle groups.

Rehabilitation does not start with the injury and finish with a return to training, but is a continuum, with no clear distinction between the rehabilitation process and a return to full competition/training. The athlete should be encouraged to be an active participant in this process.

Progression of rehabilitation

The athlete is guided through the process, progressing from one training level to the next, with the experienced clinician setting the framework for rehabilitation and being prescriptive with the athlete. There are, however, many factors influencing this, as follows:
- nature of the injury;
- length of time missed from training;
- level of the athlete pre-injury;
- aspiration/goals of the athlete;
- competition schedule and upcoming events;

- experience of the injured athlete;
- experience of the coach in dealing with the injured athlete;
- resources available to the athlete (training facilities, other support staff, funding);
- resources available to the practitioner (rehabilitation/training facilities, other sports science/sports medicine staff).

All these factors must be considered when sitting down with the athlete and coach to plan the rehabilitation phases.

Specific rehabilitation protocols

Stress fractures

The initial management of a stress fracture involves the removal of aggravating activities. Pain-free weight bearing may be necessary in some cases. A graduated return to activity is then planned and monitored.

Flexibility and strength training can begin early on, with cross-training being essential for maintaining cardiovascular fitness, for example deepwater running, swimming, biking and upper body weights.

Achilles tendonopathies

The Achilles tendon has traditionally been a difficult structure to rehabilitate. The use of an eccentric exercise programme in the rehabilitation of Achilles tendonopathies has been advocated for a number of years. There is a body of evidence to suggest that eccentric loading is more effective than concentric loading. Debate still exists, however, as to how these exercises should be undertaken:

- Fast or slow?
- Pain free or 'push into pain'?
- A progression through increased resistance, speed, volume or a combination of all three.
- Whether concentric exercises play a role in this rehabilitation process.

One such programme, as developed by Swedish orthopod Hakan Alfredsen, advocates eccentric exercise utilizing the following concepts:

- 3×15 repetitions twice daily (increased to a set of 70 eventually),
- slow eccentric lower on symptomatic leg;

- raise to the start position is done with the contralateral leg (double leg if bilateral symptoms);
- done with straight leg then bent leg;
- exercise should be painful by the last set;
- when pain free during exercise, weights are progressively added.

The above programme should be modified and incorporated into the athlete's overall training programme.

The concept of resting the tendon during the off-season carries no weight and is probably counterproductive. Best results appeared to be achieved when the tendon is allowed to settle in the first instance, before entering a strengthening programme.

As with any rehabilitation programme, all other factors need to be addressed, including biomechanical constraints, foot/ankle mobility, proximal issues, soft tissue release work and neural factors.

Hamstring strain/tear

Hamstring injuries are a regular occurrence in football and athletic sprint events. The causes are varied and may include:

- Muscle fatigue, inflexibility, poor conditioning.
- Lumbosacral spine or sacroiliac joint (SIJ) dysfunction.
- Neuromeningeal structures; either tightness or irritability.
- Superior tibio-fibular joint hypermobility.
- Muscle imbalance.
- Biomechanical factors.

This multifactorial nature of hamstring injury makes both diagnosis and treatment challenging. The following is a general rehabilitation outline, with the clinician judging which areas may need more or less attention during the process.

Rehabilitation process for grade II hamstring strain

Assessment

- Previous history of motor unit injuries.
- Site of lesion, with palpation of site above and below to gauge extent.
- History including when the pain was felt, feelings or sensation leading into the injury (including over the previous 2–3 weeks, as many athletes report a minor incident or sensation).

- Range of movement including straight leg raise (SLR), 90/90 hamstring test, hip flexion, external and internal rotation ranges.
- Resisted movements:
  - hip/knee extension with knee bent and knee straight in supine;
  - isolated hip extension in prone;
  - isolated knee extension in prone (if not too irritable).
- Lumbar spine.
- SIJ dysfunction.
- Slump (if not too irritable).

Treatment

Day 1: Ice, compression and relative rest, pain-relieving modalities.

Day 2: Continue above programme and begin pain-free continuous passive motion (CPM). (This should proceed with caution in the early phase and be pain free. It is hypothesized that CPM has a positive effect on neural dynamics and inevitable scar formation.) Spinal mobilization, soft tissue release work of structures around the pelvis and lumbar spine, light massage of the area above and below the site of the lesion.

Day 3 onwards: The speed of progression is largely dependent on symptoms. Massage to the lesion can begin with caution, continuing passive exercise through a pain-free range of movement and strengthening exercises. Begin the running programme if possible.

Running programme. Once the athlete can sit with the lumbar spine in a lordotic position, and has the ability to comfortably extend the knee to 120°, then the athlete may commence a running programme. Graham Reid, a physiotherapist with the Australian national men's field hockey programme, developed these early running programmes. They have been adapted and used successfully by many people since. The following is an example of the programme.

- Light jog.
- $3 \times 8 \times 100$ m (or 'run 100 m eight times on three occasions'; can be varied according to fitness of athlete and speed of the run).
- Accelerate for the first 30 m, hold that pace for the next 40 m, then decelerate for the last 30 m.

- Run at a comfortable pace.
- Maintain an even gait, with no limping or pain.
- Emphasis on volume and not speed.
- If one repetition feels 'not quite right', stop the session and return the next day. It is often during the next repetition that a recurrence might occur, partly as a result of neural fatigue.
- Build up to 80% pace over a number of days. (Timeframe will vary greatly, the athlete should progress at his or her own pace.)
- Once at 80%, the acceleration and deceleration phases are reduced:
  - $(30–40–30) \times 2$
  - $(25–40–25) \times 2$
  - $(20–40–20) \times 2$
  - $(15–40–15) \times 2$
  - $(10–40–10) \times 2$
- Note that the top speed of the run has not increased, but the acceleration time has decreased, thereby controlling the progression.
- From here the athlete returns to 30–40–30, but increases the speed to 85% and follows the programme through, progressing to 90%, then 95% and finally 100%.
- The number of repetitions will depend on the type of athlete and the rate of progression.
- Introduction of sports-specific events such as bend running, starting-block work, change of direction, backwards/sideways running, shuttles, chase and escape drills.

In ball sports, it is important to note that ball kicking should not commence until the athlete is running at top pace. Because of the neural factors in the hamstring lesion, it has been noted that kicking, especially for distance, creates irritability of the neural structures and compromises the accelerated running programme. There needs to be an agreement with the coach or manager to the effect that ball work may be limited, so as not to compromise the running programme, but equally, that the player does not lose the 'feel' for the ball.

Under close supervision, an accelerated return to full running, with minimal setbacks should be achieved. However, this is just an adjunct to the entire rehabilitation programme, which includes addressing relevant flexibility and strength issues (including eccentric strength programmes), hands-on therapy and causative factors.

Summary

This chapter provides a general overview of rehabilitation concepts, and some specific examples of structured programmes. It is important, however, that the clinician continues to evaluate critically these concepts and integrate them into rehabilitation programmes, whilst maintaining the core principles of the rehabilitation process.

Index